Medical disclaimer

Please do not use the information presented in this book as a substitute for the advice of a healthcare professional, certified personal trainer, or nutritionist. All information provided in this book is of a general nature and is provided for educational purposes only. No information is to be taken as medical or other health advice pertaining to any individual's specific health or medical condition. I, Edward Lord, am not engaged in providing medical or professional services. I make no guarantee regarding the accuracy, timeliness, or relevancy of any content. None of the content in this book is a diagnosis, treatment plan, or recommendation for a particular course of action regarding your health. Do not delay seeking the advice of your healthcare professional because of anything you may have read or interpreted in this book. Consult your healthcare professional before acting upon any recommendations found herein. If you experience pain at any point during exercise, please stop and consult your healthcare professional. You agree to indemnify and hold me, Edward Lord, harmless from any and all losses, liabilities, injuries, and damages resulting from decisions that you make using the content in this book. You agree that use of this information is at your own risk.

Acknowledgements

I wish to thank ExRx.net, a brilliant website that helps me to balance my weight training programs.

IMPORTANT NOTE

Numerous exercises are mentioned in this book. Unfortunately, instructions on how to perform the exercises are not provided for the simple reason that there are too many exercises. To learn how to perform the exercises, please refer to my website, **weighttraining.guide**. If you can't find an exercise on my website, please search YouTube.com. Note that the Kindle version of this book includes links to exercise descriptions on my website and YouTube.com, making life much easier. It also includes a Target Muscle Guide, a glossary, and color text and images. The Target Muscle Guide, glossary, color text and images, and links to exercise descriptions are also included in the iPhone/Android version of this book, which is available on my website.

TABLE OF CONTENTS

INTRODUCTION

Your body is special. It is a product of billions of years of evolution and consists of trillions of cells that work together to produce a single, extremely complex, durable, and adaptable biological machine. Its level of health will dictate the quality and length of your life. Its level of fitness will dictate where you can go, what you can do, and how far you can get. Its appearance will dictate people's perceptions of you and the standard of the partners that you can attract. The good news is that all of these properties — health, fitness, and appearance — can be significantly improved with training.

The purpose of this book

The purpose of this book is to give you everything you need, whether male or female, to create your best possible body. Packed with guides and training programs, it's a complete guidance and training system that contains everything necessary not only to completely transform the way your body looks but also to improve every single key component of physical fitness, from your muscular, cardiorespiratory, and functional fitness to your flexibility and body composition.

How this book is organized

This book is divided into six parts.

Part 1: Weight Training Guide

Part 1 introduces you to weight training and its benefits, goes over the details of muscle science, and reveals the fundamentals and methods of weight training. It also offers guidance on how to get started with weight training, find a gym or set up a home gym, warm up, cool down (stretch), track your progress, keep motivated, and ultimately succeed.

Part 2: Nutrition Guide

The Nutrition Guide covers all of the important elements of good nutrition, dietary management, and strategic eating. After beginning with a detailed look at all macronutrients and micronutrients, it explores calorie requirements, bulking and cutting, dietary tracking, supplementation, and nutrient timing.

Part 3: Weight training programs

In Part 3, you will find weight training programs — eight for men and eight for women. The men's programs are designed for maximum muscle and strength, whereas the women's programs are designed for maximum curves and functional strength. The eight programs include a beginner program, a minimalistic program for busy individuals, five increasingly difficult programs that cater for different levels of experience, and a "plateau buster" program designed to ensure that you never stop making progress. You can complete the training programs at any gym or at home using basic gym equipment and alternative exercises that I have provided for each program. Apart from the beginner program, all of the programs have been meticulously balanced so that you can repeat them over and over again for many years with reduced risk of developing muscular strength imbalances.

Part 4: Bodyweight, power, and plyometric workouts

Part 4 explains the fundamentals of power, plyometric, and bodyweight training, and presents power, plyometric, and equipment-free bodyweight workouts. It also gives you the tools necessary to design your own equipment-free bodyweight workouts, which you can use if you can't make it to the gym or if you go on vacation.

Part 5: Cardio Guide

The Cardio Guide begins by covering the basics of exercise physiology, the fundamentals of cardiovascular training, and the advantages, disadvantages, and applications of three types of cardio: steady-state training (SST), interval training, and functional circuit training (FCT). It then presents three cardio training programs, including one SST program with three workouts, one interval training program with three workouts (two of which are high intensity or HIIT workouts), and one FCT program with two workouts. The workouts of the three different types of cardio can of course be repeated as many times as you want to. The workouts are also interchangeable, which means that on one day you can do SST, on another day you can do HIIT, and on yet another day you can do FCT. One of the HIIT workouts follows the original Tabata protocol, which is extremely intense and intended only for experienced individuals. The Cardio Guide concludes with instructions on how to design your own FCT workouts.

Part 6: Weight Loss Guide

The Weight Loss Guide is short but very useful for anyone whose primary goal is to lose weight. It presents three steps to easier and permanent weight loss, along with a wide range of tips and tricks that can make losing weight, and keeping it off, much easier.

How to use the book to transform your body

Physical fitness can be broken down into five key components:

1. Muscular fitness (the size, strength, power, and endurance of your muscles)
2. Functional fitness (your skills as regarding agility, balance, coordination, and gait)
3. Flexibility
4. Cardiorespiratory fitness (the strength and efficiency of your heart and lungs)
5. Body composition (the amount of fat mass you have compared with fat-free mass)

This book can help you to improve all five key components of fitness, as well as transform your body's appearance.

The way you use the book will depend on your goals. If you want to develop a muscular and strong physique or a curvaceous and toned figure, start a weight training program. The weight training program will also help to improve your muscular fitness, functional fitness (because the workouts include functional exercises), flexibility (because the warmups and cooldowns include static and dynamic stretching), and body composition.

If you want to develop cardiorespiratory fitness and endurance, start a cardio training program, and mix and match the different types of workout. The cardio program will also help to improve your body composition and, if you use the FCT workouts, functional fitness.

If you want to develop all key components of physical fitness, start a weight training program *and* a cardio program. The minimalistic weight training program together with just two short cardio workouts per week should be enough to completely transform your body — from cardiorespiratory system to musculoskeletal system — and dramatically improve your weight, body composition, functional fitness, athleticism, and appearance. As to the more comprehensive and advanced weight training and cardio programs, they have the potential to give you a body similar to the one that you have always wanted!

Of course, you also have the bodyweight, power, and plyometric workouts. They, too, can help to improve your muscular fitness, functional fitness, flexibility, and body composition. Use them as and when you want to.

Ideally, you should read all of the guides before you start training. Although there's a huge amount of content to get through, the information will equip you with the strong foundational understanding of weight training, fitness, and nutrition necessary to get started on the right track, avoid injuries and mistakes, get the most out of your training, and increase your chances of success.

Please take action

A functionally stronger, healthier, fitter, and much more attractive body is within your grasp. It could be just months away. When you bought this book, you made a commitment to change. Whether you want to build an impressive physique, develop jaw-dropping curves, maximize your strength, boost your power, increase your cardiovascular endurance, lose weight, or improve your diet, this complete guidance and training system can help you to achieve your goal. All you have to do is read it and take action!

PART 1: WEIGHT TRAINING GUIDE

Chapter 1: Introduction to weight training

What is weight training?

Weight training is the practice of lifting weights, usually with the goal of personal development. Men usually do it to build muscle and strength, whereas women usually do it to develop shape and "tone". The practice involves regularly performing a list of exercises using barbells, dumbbells, and weight machines, with each exercise designed to target a different muscle group or movement pattern of the body. Over time, the amount of stress that is placed on the muscles is progressively increased, forcing the muscles to adapt by developing greater strength, size, endurance, or power. The gradual increase in stress designed to stimulate muscular development is known as **progressive overload**.

Weight training is the most common form of **strength training** (sometimes called **resistance training**). Strength training is any physical exercise that involves contracting your muscles against resistance with the aim of muscular development. Strength training can also be done using resistance bands or your own body weight.

Why do weight training?

Weight training and other forms of strength training can be performed for a number of reasons, including:

- improving your general health and fitness
- enhancing your athletic or sporting abilities
- building your muscles and strength
- sculpting a more attractive figure
- rehabilitating your limbs after an injury
- burning calories
- losing weight
- relieving stress.

How do you train?

You can train at home or in a gym, either with or without a **training partner**. Ideally, a training session should include a **warmup**, a **workout**, and a **cooldown** — all of which should take 30 to 90 minutes. The longer your workouts take, the less likely you will be to stick to them.

The warmup is very important. It prepares your mind and body for exercise, reduces your risk of injury, and gets you pumped up and ready to work out.

The cooldown, or **post-workout stretch**, involves gently stretching the muscles that you have trained, which can help to prevent stiffness and a reduction of **range of motion**.

The workout itself involves completing a list of **exercises**, of which there are numerous varieties. The types of exercise that you do depend on your goal, level of experience, and preferences. Popular exercises include the dumbbell curl, barbell bench press, and barbell squat.

For each exercise, you have to complete a certain number of **reps** and **sets**. A rep (short for **repetition**) is one complete unit of a weight training exercise, from the starting position to the point of maximum contraction and then back to the starting position. For example, you perform one rep of a dumbbell curl if you raise it to your chest and then lower it back down.

A set is a group of reps. For example, if you perform ten reps before resting, those ten reps count as one set.

The list of exercises that you perform, along with the amount of weight that you lift for each exercise and the number of sets and reps that you complete for each exercise, are defined in your **training program**.

How often must you train?

Serious lifters with lots of experience undertake five or six workouts a week, each one targeting one to three different muscle groups. However, as few as three full-body workouts per week can produce decent results.

What kinds of equipment do you need?

Common types of weight training equipment include **barbells** and **dumbbells**, which are often used in conjunction with a **bench**. More technical types of equipment include **weight machines**, which come in a variety of forms, and often incorporate seats, cables, pulleys, and levers. Barbells and dumbbells are often known as **free weights** because they are not attached to other devices and are raised and lowered freely. Unlike free weights, weight machines guide your joints through fixed patterns of motion.

Although technically not weights, **resistance bands** and your own **body weight** can also be used to develop muscles. Indeed, weight training programs often incorporate resistance band and bodyweight exercises. Resistance bands are also often used to add extra resistance to free-weight and bodyweight exercises.

You should be able to find everything you need to effectively train in a **gym**. If you're going to train at home, you will need at least a set of dumbbells, an adjustable bench, a pull-up bar, a barbell, and a **power rack** (aka **power cage**) for safety. Resistance bands and **ankle straps** can also be quite important, especially for ladies. I explain how to set up a home gym in Chapter 4, in **How to get started with weight training**.

How long does it take to see results?

Results take time, patience, and dedication, but are worth the effort. As long as you follow an effective training program that also ensures adequate rest and recovery, you should start to see evidence of an increase in strength within just days of training, and evidence of an increase in the size of your muscles (or curves) after six to eight weeks. I provide approximate figures of how much muscle the average man or woman can expect to develop per year in the next chapter, in **How quickly can you gain muscle?**

What about diet?

Good nutrition is essential for the success of your training. Your workouts will damage your muscles. Your diet must provide the raw materials necessary to repair them, as well as to build the muscles to make them stronger and less susceptible to damage. Your diet must also provide adequate fuel for your workouts. See the **Nutrition Guide** for everything you need to know about good nutrition.

What are the benefits of weight training?

Weight training comes with numerous benefits. The benefits range from improving your mental and physical health to enhancing your appearance, improving your mood, and even slowing down the aging process!

Below is a list of benefits, as divided into categories. Whenever you can't be bothered to pick up those weights at home or to hit the gym, bring your mind back to this list and remind yourself of all the positive outcomes that could result from weight training.

Physical benefits of weight training

- Build the endurance, size, strength, and power of your muscles
- Strengthen the movement patterns of your body
- Develop better balance and coordination
- Improve your athleticism and sporting performance
- Develop better body proportions and symmetry
- Improve your posture and gait
- Fix imbalances between your upper and lower body, the left and right sides of your body, and your opposing muscle groups
- Strengthen your joints, tendons, and ligaments
- Increase the density of your bones
- Make your body less prone to injury

Health benefits

- Reduce your body fat
- Reduce your cholesterol and blood fats
- Reduce high blood pressure
- Decrease your risk of heart disease
- Decrease your risk of osteoporosis
- Decrease your risk of arthritis

- Increase your metabolic rate
- Become more energetic
- Increase your endurance and flexibility
- Enhance your sleep
- Slow down the aging process

Psychological and mental benefits

- Reduce stress, anxiety, and depression
- Feel more relaxed and refreshed
- Improve your mood
- Increase your self-esteem and self-confidence
- Develop a positive self-image
- Feel a sense of achievement and empowerment
- Strengthen your willpower
- Become more disciplined
- Learn to endure pain and push your pain barrier
- Increase blood flow to your brain
- Improve your concentration and focus
- Improve your intelligence and memory
- Enhance your learning abilities

Social benefits

- Become more popular
- Command more respect and attention
- Look and feel more dominant
- Be more capable of protecting yourself and your family
- Make new friends at the gym
- Become more attractive
- Get more attention from the opposite sex

Myths of weight training and bodybuilding

Unfortunately, despite the amazing benefits of weight training, there are certain popular myths that often discourage or dissuade people from taking it up. Let's go over and dispel some of these myths.

Myth 1: If you stop exercising, your muscles will turn into fat

This is impossible. Muscle tissue and fat tissue are two completely different things. One cannot turn into the other. If you stop training, you will gradually lose the muscle, shape, and strength, but you will put on weight only if you eat more calories than you burn.

Myth 2: It takes a lot of time and effort to see good results

As long as you do the three main things — train, eat, and rest — correctly, you can experience remarkable results within just six months, training one hour a day and four days a week. That's just four hours a week! Your friends and family should start to notice a difference after just eight or so weeks. See **How quickly can you gain muscle?** in Chapter 2.

Myth 3: Weight training decreases your flexibility

If you train correctly, making sure to use proper form and put your joints through their full range of motion, you will likely improve your flexibility, not lose it. However, loss of flexibility is possible in three instances:

1. If you consistently lift heavy weights using a partial range of motion.
2. If you overdevelop one muscle group relative to its opposing muscle group.
3. If you damage a muscle, joint, tendon, or ligament while training.

These three instances can easily be avoided by utilizing the full range of motion, stretching your muscles after each workout, following a balanced training program, and being careful when you train.

Myth 4: Weight training damages your joints

Actually, weight training is an effective way of strengthening your joints. Other forms of physical exercise, such as running and jumping, actually place far more stress on your joints than weight training does. As long as you perform weight training exercises correctly, using proper form and technique, and adhere to safety recommendations, weight training will strengthen the ligaments that hold your joints together, thus making them more stable and less susceptible to injury.

Myth 5: Weight training makes women look masculine

This is one of the most discouraging of the myths of weight training. It's regrettable because weight training can help women to increase energy levels, reduce fat, improve muscle tone, enhance their curves, create a better body shape, reduce the risk of developing certain diseases (for example, osteoporosis), and even slow down the aging process — all without making them look masculine! It's actually very difficult for women to achieve that big, bulky, masculine look because they lack testosterone, possessing only one-tenth of the amount that men do. The only way that women can achieve the bulky, masculine look is if they train like crazy and use steroids.

Chapter 2: Muscle science

Muscle names

Why you should learn muscle names

If you are going to take up weight training, you should familiarize yourself with your **musculoskeletal system**, or at least learn the names of the major muscles that you will be training (Figure 2.1). Being familiar with your muscles and how they function will help you to choose the right exercises, practice proper form when you train, and better target your muscles. If you know muscle names, you will also be able to communicate your goals to others more clearly and efficiently.

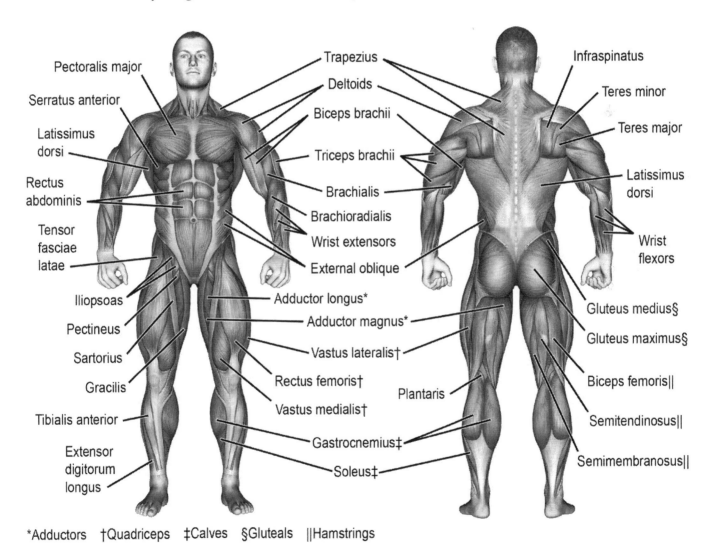

*Adductors †Quadriceps ‡Calves §Gluteals ||Hamstrings

Figure 2.1. The superficial muscles of the human body, showing both anterior and posterior views. The muscles are of course the same in both men and women.

Depending on whom you ask, there are between 640 and 700 named muscles in the human body, which doesn't include the hundreds of smaller muscles that have not been named. However, for our purposes, we only need to learn the names of the major muscles, most of which are labeled in Figure 2.1.

How to memorize muscle names

To help yourself memorize muscle names, identify them in your own body, and try to flex them. You could also write them down, create flash cards, draw a mind map, or even make up a song. I found that the best way to remember muscle names is to draw and label them, as well as describe them to other people.

Muscle naming conventions

Muscle names are actually quite interesting. Usually derived from Latin, a muscle's name often tells you something about the muscle, such as its location, origin, number of origins, insertion, size, shape, direction, or function.

Location

Many muscle names indicate the muscle's location. For example, the tibialis anterior is named after the part of the bone to which it is attached (the anterior portion of the tibia), and the names of the brachialis and brachioradialis muscles tell you that they are located in the arm because the word *bracchium* means "arm" in Latin.

Number of origins

Muscles are usually attached to two bones. One end of the muscle attaches to one bone and the other end attaches to another. Traditionally, the proximal end of a muscle (the end of the muscle that is closest to the head) is known as its **origin**, whereas the distal end of a muscle (the end of the muscle that is farthest from the head) is known as its **insertion** (Figure 2.2).

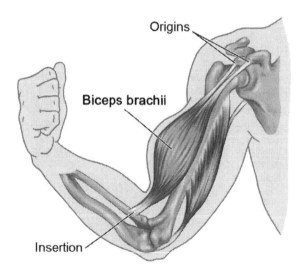

Figure 2.2. The two origins and the insertion of the biceps brachii.

A number of muscles have more than one origin, and this is sometimes expressed in their names. For example, a biceps muscle has two origins, a triceps muscle has three origins, and a quadriceps muscle has four origins.

Size

Many muscles located close together in a specific region of the body are named after their size. For example, in the buttock region, you have the gluteus minimus (small), gluteus medius (medium), and gluteus maximus (large). Longus (longest) and brevis (shortest) are other common suffixes added to muscle names.

Shape

Some muscles are named after shapes. For example, the shoulder muscle, more properly known as the deltoid, has a Delta-like or triangular shape; the trapezius has a trapezoid shape; the serratus anterior has a serrated or saw-toothed shape; and the rhomboid major has a rhomboidal or diamond-like shape.

Direction

The terms rectus (parallel), transverse (perpendicular), and oblique (at an angle) in muscle names tell you the angle in which the muscle's fibers run relative to the midline of the body. For example, in the abdominal region, the fibers of the rectus abdominis run parallel with the midline, the fibers of the transverse abdominis run perpendicular relative to the midline, and the fibers of the external oblique run at an angle relative to the midline.

Function

Muscles are also sometimes named after their function or action. Terms such as flexor, extensor, abductor, and adductor are added to muscle names to indicate the kind of movement that they generate. For example, the wrist flexors flex the wrist, the wrist extensors extend the wrist, and the adductor magnus adducts the thigh (pulls it towards the midline).

Muscle structure

Your muscles make up nearly half of your body weight. They are composed of over 75% water; the rest is mostly protein. Being familiar with skeletal muscle structure, especially the characteristics of the different muscle fiber types, is important because it will help you to understand how to develop the different muscle properties: size, strength, endurance, and power.

The three types of muscle

There are three types of muscle in your body, each with a different muscle structure:

1. Cardiac (striated, involuntary)
2. Smooth (non-striated, involuntary)
3. Skeletal (striated, voluntary)

Cardiac muscle appears striated under a microscope, and can be found in the walls of your heart. Triggered by impulses from your **autonomic nervous system**, it contracts involuntarily and is responsible for pumping your blood around your body.

Smooth muscle appears smooth (non-striated) under a microscope, and can be found in the walls of hollow organs throughout your body, such as your bladder. It allows these organs to expand and contract as required. Smooth muscle can also be found in your eyes, blood vessels, and digestive tract. In your eyes, it changes the shape of your lenses to bring objects into focus; in the walls of your blood vessels, it contracts and relaxes to move blood through the vessels; and in your digestive tract, it is responsible for producing the peristaltic movements that push food through your digestive system. Like cardiac muscle, smooth muscle contractions are involuntary, triggered by impulses from your autonomic nervous system.

Skeletal muscle appears striated under a microscope. Skeletal muscles attach to your bones via tendons, and move your bones by contracting and relaxing in response to voluntary messages sent by your **somatic nervous system**. Skeletal muscles are responsible for locomotion, and changing and maintaining your body posture. Together with your bones, they make up your **musculoskeletal system**.

Skeletal muscle structure

Skeletal muscles (Figure 2.3) are composed of long, cylindrical cells called **muscle fibers** (or **myocytes**), which are approximately the width of a human hair in diameter (50 to 100 micrometers). They are among the largest cells in the human body, ranging from a few centimeters to one meter in length.

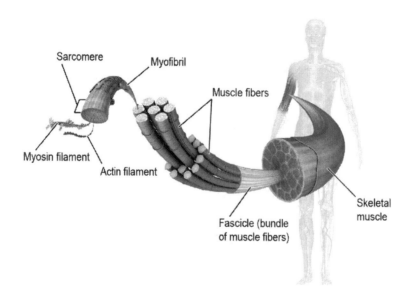

Figure 2.3. A breakdown of the structure of skeletal muscles right down to the contractile filaments actin and myosin. The filaments form units called sarcomeres, which, stacked end to end, make myofibrils, the strands within muscle fibers. Bundles of muscle fibers produce fascicles, which in turn make up skeletal muscles.

Muscle fibers have more than one nucleus, and are composed of cylindrical strands called **myofibrils**, each one approximately one micrometer in diameter. The myofibrils are in turn composed of filaments of the proteins **actin** and **myosin**, which repeat in units known as **sarcomeres**.

Sarcomeres are the basic functional units of muscle fibers. As you will soon learn, they form the basic machinery necessary for muscle contraction. Sarcomeres are also responsible for the striated appearance of skeletal muscle tissue.

Types of muscle fiber

There are three types of muscle fiber:

1. Type I (oxidative slow-twitch)
2. Type IIa (oxidative fast-twitch)
3. Type IIb (glycolytic fast-twitch)

Table 2.1 summarizes their characteristics.

	Type I	**Type IIa**	**Type IIb**
Diameter	Narrow	Medium	Wide
Contraction speed	Slow	Moderately fast	Fast
Power produced	Small	Moderate	Large
Activity used for	Aerobic	Long-term anaerobic	Short-term anaerobic
Endurance	High	Moderate	Low
Max. duration of use	Hours	Less than 30 min	Less than 1 min

Table 2.1. The characteristics of the three different types of muscle fiber.

Type I fibers are narrow in diameter and contract relatively slowly, which is why they are also called **slow-twitch muscle fibers**. Type I fibers are used for low-intensity, aerobic activities, such as jogging and lifting light weights. They have a high endurance level and therefore do not tire easily.

Type IIb fibers are wide in diameter and contract relatively rapidly, which is why they are also called **fast-twitch muscle fibers**. They are used for high-intensity, anaerobic activities, such as sprinting and lifting heavy weights, and can generate relatively high levels of tension. Type IIb fibers have low endurance, which means that they tire easily.

18

Type IIa fibers are another type of fast-twitch muscle fiber. Their characteristics fall in between those of Type I and Type IIb fibers.

Type IIa and Type IIb fibers increase in size more readily and at a faster rate than do Type I fibers.

Muscle fiber types and muscle function

Each of your skeletal muscles contains a mixture of the three types of muscle fiber, thus providing each muscle with the ability to produce an increasing amount of force, from low to high. When you lift light weights, your Type I fibers do most of the work. If you increase the amount of weight being lifted, an increasing number of Type IIa fibers will be recruited to help with the lifting. If you lift very heavy weights, virtually all Type I, Type IIa, and Type IIb fibers will be recruited.

How the different types of muscle fiber affect muscle properties

You were born with a specific ratio of muscle fiber types in each muscle. As the three types of muscle fiber have different characteristics, the ratio dictates how much strength or endurance each muscle has: Muscles that contain more Type I fibers will have more endurance than muscles that contain more Type IIb fibers. Conversely, muscles that contain more Type IIb fibers will have more strength than muscles that contain more Type I fibers. Since Type IIa and Type IIb fibers increase in size more readily and at a faster rate than do Type I fibers, the ratio of muscle fibers also dictates how large the muscle can grow.

How muscles work

Motor units

Your skeletal muscles are controlled by your **somatic nervous system**. Muscle contractions are activated by nerve cells called **motor neurons** (Figure 2.4). A single motor neuron may stimulate between one and several hundred muscle fibers. Some motor neurons activate Type I fibers, whereas others activate Type IIa or Type IIb fibers. A motor neuron and the fibers that it stimulates are collectively called a **motor unit**. If a motor neuron fires, it activates *all* of the muscle fibers in its motor unit.

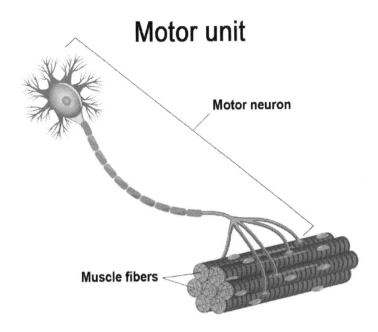

Figure 2.4. A motor neuron and the muscle fibers that it activates, which collectively make a motor unit.

How motor units are recruited for contraction

The contraction of a single muscle is often coordinated by groups of motor units. The number of motor units involved in the contraction depends on the amount of load. If the load is light, a relatively small number of Type I motor units will be recruited. As the load increases, more Type I motor units will be called into action, and then Type IIa and Type IIb motor units, until all of the muscle's motor units are utilized. *This means that the only way to stimulate the entire muscle is to work with weights that are personally very heavy.*

How muscles contract

As mentioned above, muscle fibers are composed of cylindrical strands called **myofibrils**, which are in turn composed of filaments of the proteins **actin** and **myosin**. The filaments, known as **myofilaments**, repeat in units called **sarcomeres**. The two ends of each sarcomere are marked by a **Z disc**.

Sarcomeres are the basic functional units of muscle fibers. If you understand how sarcomeres function, you will understand how muscles work.

Put simply, when an impulse from a motor neuron reaches the muscle fiber, it creates chemical changes that cause the actin filaments to slide along the myosin filaments, which shortens the length of the sarcomere and thus changes the length and shape of the muscle fiber (Figure 2.5). Once the stimulation stops, the actin and myosin filaments move apart, and the sarcomere (and thus the muscle fiber) returns to its resting length and shape.

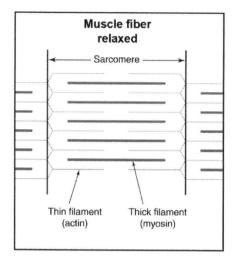 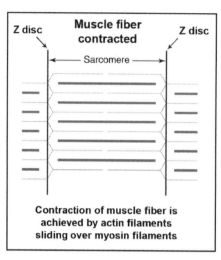 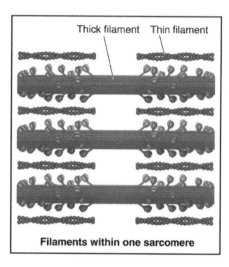

Figure 2.5. Muscle fiber contraction. Muscle fibers contract at the level of the sarcomere when thin actin filaments slide over thick myosin filaments as a result of chemical changes initiated by an impulse from a motor neuron.

More specifically, the thick myosin filaments possess protruding heads that can bind to the thin actin filaments. When an impulse hits the muscle fiber, the protruding heads of the myosin filaments bind to the actin filaments, after which the myosin filaments undergo a change in shape. The change in shape cocks the protruding heads of the myosin filaments, which pulls the actin filaments inwards. Since the actin filaments are anchored to the ends of the sarcomere (the Z discs), the sarcomere shortens in length. All of the sarcomeres in the muscle fiber shorten at the same time, producing the action that we call **contraction**.

How muscles grow

What is neuromuscular adaptation?

When you first start weight training, the nerve pathways that serve your motor units undergo changes to become more efficient, thus improving your ability to recruit muscle fibers. This is known as **neuromuscular adaptation**, and is responsible for most of the gains in strength that you experience during the first six to eight weeks of training. The gains in strength start to occur within just days and are due solely to this process of your body "learning" to use your existing muscles more efficiently. Only then does your body invest in building extra muscle.

What is hypertrophy?

As long as you stick to an effective training program, your muscles will start to grow after the initial neuromuscular adaptation phase (six to eight weeks). The scientific name for the increase in size of your muscles is **hypertrophy**. Hypertrophy occurs due to an increase in the *diameter* of your muscle fibers; it does not occur due to an increase in the *number* of your muscle fibers.

Since Type IIa and Type IIb muscle fibers increase in size more readily and at a faster rate than Type I fibers do, the increase in muscle mass and strength is mainly due to the increase in size of Type II fibers. And since Type II fibers are recruited only when you lift personally heavy weights, if you want to build muscle or curves, you have to lift personally heavy weights.

How does hypertrophy occur?

When you train, the filaments of actin and myosin that control muscle-fiber contraction sustain **microdamage**. Damage also occurs to connective tissues. It's this microdamage that causes post-workout pain and soreness.

While you rest, the connective tissues and contractile filaments are repaired with new proteins. Extra filaments are added to prevent future damage, which increases the diameter of the muscle fibers and therefore increases the diameter and strength of the muscle. The increase in muscle fiber diameter is accompanied by an increase in other cellular properties, such as **sarcoplasm**.

Sarcoplasm is the **cytoplasm** of the muscle fiber — that is, the gel-like substance within the muscle fiber, along with its **organelles**. It differs from the cytoplasm of other types of body cell by containing unusually large amounts of **myoglobin** and **glycogen granules** (**glycosomes**). Myoglobin is a protein that carries oxygen, and glycosomes are the muscle fiber's primary source of energy. The increase in the amount of sarcoplasm therefore makes sense: Larger muscle fibers need more oxygen and energy.

Sarcoplasmic hypertrophy vs myofibrillar hypertrophy

Hypertrophy is often divided into two types:

1. Sarcoplasmic
2. Myofibrillar

Myofibrillar hypertrophy refers specifically to an increase in the number and diameter of myofibrils, which occurs due to the increase in the size and number of contractile filaments. Sarcoplasmic hypertrophy, on the other hand, refers specifically to an increase in the volume of sarcoplasm.

Due to the increase in size and number of contractile filaments, myofibrillar hypertrophy is accompanied by an increase in strength and a small increase in muscular size, whereas sarcoplasmic hypertrophy is accompanied by an increase in size and a small increase in strength.

These two types of hypertrophy do not occur completely independently of one another: Depending on how you train, you can experience either a large increase in sarcoplasm with a small increase in contractile proteins, a large increase in contractile proteins with a small increase in sarcoplasm, or a relatively balanced increase in both. Sarcoplasmic hypertrophy is more dominant in the muscles of bodybuilders, who train for muscle size, whereas myofibrillar hypertrophy is more dominant in the muscles of powerlifters and Olympic weightlifters, who train for strength and power.

Different types of training affect how muscles grow. You will learn how to train for each type of hypertrophy and thus either develop muscular size, strength, or both in Chapter 3, in **How many sets and reps should you do?**

How quickly can you gain muscle?

Building muscle or curves takes time, patience, and dedication, but is worth the effort. According to one popular model of muscle growth presented by Lyle McDonald of BodyRecomposition.com, the average rates of muscle gain that men can expect following proper training and nutrition vary depending on years of training experience. In his first year of proper training and nutrition, the average man can expect to gain between 20 and 25 pounds of muscle, which equates to approximately two pounds of muscle mass per month. As illustrated in Table 2.2, the rate of muscle gain then starts to plummet.

Years of proper training	Potential rate of muscle growth per year	
	Men	Women
1	20–25 lb (2 lb/month)	10–12.5 lb (1 lb/month)
2	10–12 lb (1 lb/month)	5–6 lb (0.5 lb/month)
3	5–6 lb (0.5 lb/month)	2.5–3 lb (0.25 lb/month)
4+	2–3 lb (not worth calculating)	1–1.5 lb (not worth calculating)

Table 2.2. Average rate of potential male and female muscle growth per year.

Women who do not take steroids can expect to achieve half of the values in Table 2.2 — that is, 10 to 12.5 pounds of muscle gain in the first year of proper training and nutrition. One of the main reasons is that women tend to have far less testosterone, which is, of course, an important hormone for muscle growth.

Age is not mentioned in the model, but is a factor: Mature individuals will probably see less of a gain than young individuals.

McDonald makes the point that a man who has been following a poor training program for four years and therefore has gained very little muscle mass may still be able to gain 20 to 25 pounds of muscle in his fifth year of training if he starts training and eating properly. Likewise, a woman who has been following a poor training program for four years may still be able to gain 10 to 12.5 pounds of muscle in her fifth year of training if she starts training and eating properly.

If the values in the table are summed, it suggests that the average man can expect to gain between 37 and 46 pounds of lean muscle mass in his first four years of proper training and nutrition, after which he can expect to gain only two to three pounds of muscle mass in each subsequent year of training. The average woman, on the other hand, can expect to gain between 18.5 and 23 pounds of lean muscle mass in her first four years of proper training and nutrition, after which she can expect to gain only one to two pounds of muscle mass in each subsequent year of training.

Genetic factors that limit muscle growth

Although everybody can use weight training to dramatically increase the size of their muscles or curves, there are some genetically determined factors that limit how much and how fast muscles/curves can be developed. These include:

1. the number of fibers in your muscles
2. the ratio of Type I to Type II fibers in your muscles
3. your body type
4. your hormonal balance, especially your testosterone level.

Let's look at each of these limitations individually.

The number of fibers in your muscles

You were born with a specific number of muscle fibers per motor unit, and, unfortunately, there is nothing you can do to increase the number. If you have an above-average number, you will have the potential to gain more strength and size than someone with an average number of muscle fibers. Conversely, if you have a below-average number, you will lack the potential to gain as much strength and size as someone who has an average number of muscle fibers.

The ratio of Type I to Type II fibers in your muscles

As you're aware, there are three types of muscle fiber: Type I, Type IIa, and Type IIb. Type I fibers are better suited for endurance, whereas Type II fibers are better suited for size, strength, speed, and power.

Each skeletal muscle in your body has a mixture of fiber types. The ratio of fiber types in each muscle, which is largely genetically determined, dictates your muscles', and therefore your, abilities. For example, if you have a high ratio of Type II to Type I fibers, you will be able to gain muscle mass relatively quickly and have the potential to do well in sports that require a lot of strength, speed, and power. On the other hand, if you have a high ratio of Type I to Type II fibers, you will make slower gains in muscular size, and have the potential to do well at sports that require endurance.

While it is not possible to change your ratio of fiber types, it *is* possible to change the properties of some Type II fibers and make them more like Type I fibers. With regular aerobic training, Type IIa and Type IIb

24

fibers can become more aerobic, develop greater capacity for endurance, and be more like Type I fibers. However, it is not possible for Type I fibers to assume the characteristics of Type II fibers.

Body type

Generally speaking, there are three main body types (aka **somatotypes**): **ectomorph**, **endomorph**, and **mesomorph** (Figure 2.6). Each somatotype has a different potential to add muscle and fat.

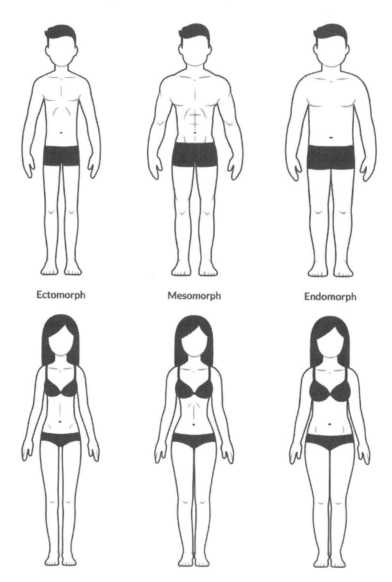

Figure 2.6. The characteristics of the three main body types (somatotypes), ectomorph (left), mesomorph (center), and endomorph (right).

Ectomorphs are lean and thin. They lack bulk and possess low levels of body fat. They also have long limbs, narrow shoulders and hips, and a fast metabolism that makes it difficult to gain muscle or fat. The majority of professional basketball players are ectomorphs.

Endomorphs have a naturally stocky and rounded body with wide shoulders and wide hips. They have an even distribution of fat, and gain muscle and fat easily. Many football players and wrestlers are endomorphs, as are many strongmen.

Mesomorphs have a naturally athletic build with wide shoulders and narrow hips. They gain muscle readily and find it relatively easy to lose fat. Mesomorphs therefore make the best bodybuilders.

Most people are a mixture of these body types, but tend to lean towards one more strongly than the others. Whichever one you are, don't worry; you can still achieve great results. Just follow the guidelines of good nutrition and effective training.

Level of testosterone

Testosterone and growth hormone (GH) play an important role in the growth of muscle (hypertrophy). If you have high levels of testosterone and GH, you will respond to training more readily and make greater gains in muscle and strength. Since men possess ten times more testosterone than women do, hypertrophy is easier for men. The only way that women can achieve muscular growth near the same level as men is by taking additional testosterone in the form of anabolic steroids, which, of course, is not recommended.

How to naturally increase testosterone

Here are some ways in which men can naturally increase their testosterone level or at least ensure that testosterone production is optimal.

Lose weight

If you're overweight, try to lose weight. The more body fat you have, the more influence **estrogen** will have on your body, and estrogen is detrimental to testosterone. On the other hand, the more muscle you have, the more testosterone you will have.

Train hard and for a short period of time

Short, intense training with heavy weights has a proven positive effect on increasing testosterone. That's unlike aerobic exercises, which have been shown to have negative or no effect on testosterone production. Short, intense training, including performing reps to failure, will stress your body, and the more you stress your body, the more testosterone will be released. The best way to stress your body is by concentrating on major compound exercises, such as the barbell deadlift and the barbell squat, which simultaneously work multiple joints and muscle groups.

Reduce stress

When you're under a lot of stress, your body releases high levels of the stress hormone **cortisol**, which actually blocks the effects of testosterone.

Boost your intake of BCAAs

Branched-chain amino acids (BCAAs) promote higher testosterone and growth hormone levels, particularly when taken in conjunction with weight training. You can buy BCAAs in supplemental form, as well as find them in high concentrations in dairy products, especially quality cheeses and whey proteins.

Eat healthy fats

Healthy fats are essential for testosterone production. Therefore, make sure that you get enough healthy fats in your diet. By "healthy", I mean not only mono- and polyunsaturated fats but also saturated fats, which are healthy in moderation.

Eat less sugar

Testosterone levels decrease after you eat sugar, which is likely because the sugar leads to a high insulin level, another factor leading to low testosterone.

Garlic

Garlic has been proven to elevate testosterone levels. It contains a compound called **allicin**, which scientific studies have proven to simultaneously decrease cortisol and raise testosterone.

Get some zinc

The mineral zinc is important for testosterone production, and supplementing your diet for as little as six weeks has been shown to cause a marked improvement in testosterone among men with low levels. **ZMA** is a good example of a popular zinc-containing supplement.

Chapter 3: Fundamentals and methods of weight training

Guidelines and principles

Before diving into training, it's very important to understand the guidelines and principles of weight training, as presented below. They are essential if you want to start on the right track, get the most out of your training, avoid mistakes, reduce your risk of injury, and achieve your goal as quickly as possible.

The formula for success

The general formula for success in weight training is very straightforward:

1. Train
2. Eat
3. Rest
4. Repeat

As long as you follow an effective training program, consume the right amounts of the right nutrients, get adequate rest to allow your body to recover (which should be incorporated into your training program), and keep repeating this sequence, you should see positive results.

Progressive overload

The weight training exercises that you perform will place stress on your muscles, which will force them to adapt. Depending on the type of training that you do, the adaptation can be an increase in muscular size, strength, endurance, or power. To ensure continual adaptation and progress, you have to gradually increase the amount of stress that you place on your muscles. Depending on your goal (size, strength, endurance, or power), the increase in stress can be:

- an increase in resistance (the amount of weight that you lift)
- an increase in the number of exercises, sets, or reps that you perform
- a decrease in the amount of time that you rest between sets and exercises.

The gradual increase in stress designed to stimulate continual muscular development is known as **progressive overload**. It is one of the primary principles of weight training and an essential element of your training program. The training programs in this book implement progressive overload safely and effectively.

Safety always comes first

Weight training can be dangerous. Not only can you drop weights on your feet and trip over rogue dumbbells but you can also damage joints, tear ligaments, and impinge nerves if you don't exercise properly or if you fail to follow important guidelines or principles. Even worse, if you are not careful, you can hurt someone else. With that in mind, always remember that your main priority when working out is not to develop your muscles or curves but rather to stay safe and injury-free. See **Safety always comes first**, at the end of this chapter, for safety tips and advice.

Always warm up before, and cool down after, a workout

An important element of practicing safety is making sure that you always warm up before you work out. Warming up reduces your likelihood of sustaining an injury by preparing your mind and body for exercise. The recommended procedure of warming up is presented in Chapter 4, in **How to warm up**.

Cooling down after a workout, which simply involves gently stretching the muscles that you have trained, is also important for safety. The procedure, which is covered in Chapter 4, in **How to cool down**, helps to keep your muscles, tendons, and ligaments strong, thus decreasing your risk of damaging them in the future. The post-workout stretch also helps to prevent a reduction in the range of motion of your joints, which may occur if you consistently exercise using a partial range of motion.

Practice proper form and technique

Each exercise that you perform has an ideal method of execution. Performing the exercise using the ideal method of execution ensures that the proper muscle groups are activated, the full range of motion is achieved, and the proper movement pattern is strengthened — all of which ensure maximum results. Sticking to the ideal method of execution also minimizes the risk of injury and prevents a reduction in your joints' range of motion. Therefore, always be strict when it comes to form and technique. The proper form of most of the exercises mentioned in this book is covered in the **Exercise Database** on my website:

http://weighttraining.guide/category/exercises/

General tips for proper form and technique

- Before trying a new exercise, study its details closely.
- Practice execution of the exercise using light weights.
- Perform every rep using the full range of motion without locking out your joints, which will help to prevent joint damage.
- Maintain full control of the weight at all times. Do not swing the weight because momentum will take over, your target muscle(s) will cease to be the focus, and you will endanger your joints.
- Visualize the contraction and relaxation of your target muscle. This will reinforce the mind–body connection, which will give you better control of your body. It's also believed to produce better results.
- Watch experienced gym-goers, and don't be afraid to ask for advice.

Perform reps at the right tempo

An important element of practicing proper form is performing reps at the right tempo or speed. Unless training to develop power, do reps relatively slowly and deliberately. Muscle-fiber growth is closely correlated with the amount of time a muscle is put under tension. Fast, intense reps do increase strength and power, but they do not lead to as much gains in muscle mass and endurance as do slower, more deliberate reps. The ideal rep tempo is different depending on whether you are training for strength, size, endurance, or power. The different tempos are discussed below, in **How many sets and reps should you do?**

Maintain equal focus on concentric and eccentric rep phases

Generally speaking, reps are divided into two phases:

1. Concentric/Positive (for example, when, during a dumbbell curl, you raise the dumbbell to your chest)
2. Eccentric/Negative (when you lower the dumbbell back to the starting position)

One complete rep goes through the joint's full **range of motion**.

Many beginners focus only on the concentric phase of the movement because that's when they strain against the weight. However, it's now well known that the eccentric phase actually has more muscle-splitting potential than does the concentric phase, which means that the part when you lower the dumbbell is actually more important for building muscle than the part when you lift it! Therefore, to get the best results, focus on both phases of every rep.

Don't forget to breathe

Breathing is something you will almost certainly have to work on. Get into the habit of breathing properly from the outset so that you will not have to try to fix improper breathing habits in the future. The general rule is to inhale during the eccentric phase of the rep and exhale during the concentric phase. For example, if doing the barbell squat, inhale as you squat and exhale as you stand back up. Try not to hold your breath.

Sometimes, such as when deadlifting or squatting a very heavy weight, you can't help but to hold your breath. There is even a technique to it, known as the **Valsalva maneuver**, which involves taking a deep breath and attempting to exhale while closing your airway. This produces internal pressure that supports your core and helps you to generate power during the lift. If you use the Valsalva maneuver, try not to hold your breath for longer than a couple of seconds.

Flush your muscles

Unless you're performing supersets (explained later in this chapter, in **Advanced methods of training**) or following a circuit training program, perform all exercises for one muscle group before moving on to the exercises of the next muscle group. In other words, focus your attention on one muscle group at a time. This allows you to "flush" each muscle group — that is, boost the blood flow to that area of the body, giving the area a good "pump", and ensuring that it gets adequate oxygen and nutrients. Flushing is one of the classic principles of weight training and bodybuilding.

Exercise large muscle groups before small ones

Unless you are following a pre-exhaustion protocol (which will be covered below, in **Advanced methods of training**), perform exercises that target your large muscle groups first. This principle will be prewritten into any decent training program. The reason is that small muscle groups tend to assist large ones, and if you tire the small ones first, they will not be able to offer proper assistance to the large muscle groups. As a result, you will limit your ability to overload your large muscle groups. For example, your triceps brachii assist your chest when you perform the bench press. If you train your triceps brachii before you train your chest, you will not be able to do much lifting with your chest.

Large muscle groups include:

- Quadriceps (rectus femoris, vastus lateralis, vastus medialis, and vastus intermedius)
- Gluteals (gluteus maximus, gluteus medius, and gluteus minimus)
- Hamstrings (biceps femoris, semitendinosus, and semimembranosus)
- Back (latissimus dorsi, trapezius, erector spinae, teres major, rhomboids, infraspinatus, and teres minor)
- Chest (pectoralis major, pectoralis minor, and serratus anterior)
- Shoulders (anterior deltoid, lateral deltoid, and posterior deltoid)

Small muscle groups include:

- Abdominals (rectus abdominis, internal oblique, and external oblique)
- Calves (soleus and gastrocnemius)
- Triceps brachii
- Biceps brachii
- Forearms (brachioradialis, wrist flexors, and wrist extensors)

Prioritize weak areas of a muscle group

Different exercises can target different areas of a muscle group. For example, both the barbell bench press and the reverse-grip barbell bench press target your pectoralis major (chest); however, the barbell bench press mainly targets your lower (sternal) pectoralis major, whereas the reverse-grip barbell bench press mainly targets your upper (clavicular) pectoralis major. If your upper chest is lagging, start with the reverse-grip barbell bench press before moving on to the barbell bench press.

Follow a balanced training program

When choosing a training program, it's very important to pick one that balances movement patterns in accordance with recommended muscle strength ratios. Otherwise, in the long run, you could develop strength imbalances between opposing muscle groups, which could lead to bad posture, joint instability, muscle tightness, pain, and injury. For example, most men train their internal shoulder rotators (pectoralis major, anterior deltoid, latissimus dorsi, teres major, and subscapularis) much more than they train their external shoulder rotators (posterior deltoid, infraspinatus, and teres minor). As a result, the tightness of their internal shoulder rotators can in time pull their shoulders forward, giving them a "caveman" posture!

To make the matter worse, their rotator cuffs, which keep their shoulder joints in place, can become compromised, leading to joint instability, impingement, and pain. The strategy that I used to balance the men's and women's training programs in this book is explained in the men's and women's respective training program overviews.

Do not neglect your legs

Many men interested in building muscle focus on their upper body much more than on their lower body. Some even completely forego training their legs! This is a very bad idea. The human body is a system. If one half is trained, the other half must also be trained to preserve balance, symmetry, and proportions. What's more, if you do not give your legs equal attention:

1. your weak legs will limit the abilities or your upper body. Your legs act as your base, and without a strong base, you will not be able to do much with your upper body
2. you'll experience slower and limited overall muscle gains. The reason is that your legs house your largest muscle groups, and when you exercise large muscle groups, your body releases more anabolic hormones, which promote body-wide muscular development. This means that if you want big arms, you must train your legs.

Do not neglect your upper body

Just as some men neglect their legs, some women neglect their upper body, especially their chest and back. The reason usually is that they are afraid of looking too muscular. Women already naturally have a stronger lower body than an upper body. This is their natural balance. However, by neglecting their upper body, they can break that balance.

By giving the upper body the attention that it deserves, women can maintain their natural balance, as well as develop more ideal proportions and features. For example, tightening the back muscles and posterior deltoids will keep the shoulders back, building the chest muscles will raise the breasts, and broadening the shoulders will make the waist look thinner — all without looking too muscular. The additional upper-body muscle will also help to increase metabolism, which burns more calories and increases energy levels. What's more, the stronger upper body will help to train the lower body.

Cultivate a strong core

The word "core" refers to all of the muscles in your torso, especially your abdominals, obliques, spinal erectors, and various other deep muscles that attach to your spine and pelvis. Having a strong core is very important because your core muscles work together to stabilize your body during lifts and movements, as well as to transfer energy from one side of your body to the other, or from your lower body to your upper body. Your core is also where you generate most of your power. As such, it can be considered your body's **power base**.

By training your core, you can increase strength and stability throughout your body, build power, promote more efficient movements, and improve balance and coordination — all of which can improve performance and reduce the risk of injury. Therefore, ensure that your training program incorporates effective core training.

Note that isolating your abs with the crunch does not count as effective core training! Proper core training involves performing major compound and functional exercises that simultaneously engage multiple core muscles. Such exercises include the squat, deadlift, clean and jerk, lunge, weighted push-up, pull-up, plank, wheel rollout, bicycle crunch, hanging leg and hip raise, Russian twist, cable wood chop, and lying side hip raise. All of the training programs in this book incorporate effective core training.

Strengthen all primal movement patterns

Your body is designed to move in certain key ways, known as **primal movement patterns**. They are:

1. Squat
2. Lunge (forward, sideways, and backward)
3. Flex/Extend the hips
4. Twist (and resist twisting)
5. Pull (horizontal and vertical)
6. Push (horizontal and vertical)
7. Gait (walk, run, and jump)

You use these movements every day of your life. For example, you squat as you sit down, you lunge over puddles, you bend at the hips to get out of bed or to pick something up, and you twist whenever you reach for the side drawer under your desk or throw a ball for your dog to fetch. The seven primal movement patterns are used in different combinations in everyday activities, and are especially important for athleticism and sporting performance. It's therefore very important to perform exercises that strengthen these movement patterns. In so doing, you will develop **functional strength** — the kind of strength that not only improves your overall fitness and athleticism but is also useful in everyday life.

Unfortunately, many training programs focus solely on training muscles, not movement patterns. You are asked to perform certain exercises for each muscle group. Often, the exercises are isolation exercises, which strengthen movement patterns that are of no use outside of the gym. For example, the dumbbell fly movement pattern is only useful if you want to give people tight hugs! The good news is that the training programs in this book incorporate effective compound and functional exercises that work to strengthen all of your body's primal movement patterns, thus improving your overall fitness and athleticism, and helping you to get the most out of your time at the gym.

Incorporate unilateral training

An important element of developing functional strength is to perform **unilateral exercises** (exercises that allow you to train one side of your body at a time). Most daily activities are unilateral, so it makes sense to include exercises that strengthen unilateral movement patterns. All dumbbell exercises and many cable and machine exercises can be performed unilaterally, so you should alternate, sometimes doing them bilaterally and other times performing them unilaterally. This will also add variation to your program, which will keep you engaged.

Unilateral exercises have other benefits:

- Since they put you off balance, they force the recruitment of more stabilizer muscles, especially in your core.
- They can be used to fix issues with symmetry and contralateral muscle strength (that is, differences in strength between the right and left sides of your body).

To ensure the strengthening of unilateral movement patterns, unilateral exercises have been included in all of the training programs in this book. When performing a unilateral exercise, always start with your weak side, and never complete more reps with your strong side. This will allow your weak side to catch up.

Types of exercise

There are literally thousands of weight training exercises and exercise variations. All of the exercises can be categorized into two groups: **isolation** and **compound**. The same exercises can also be divided into **pull** and **push** categories, or **primary**, **assistance**, and **auxiliary** categories. All of these categories are explained below. I also define **aerobic** and **anaerobic** exercises.

Isolation and compound exercises

Probably the most common exercise classification scheme is to divide them into isolation and compound categories.

Isolation exercises are those that involve the movement of only one joint (or one pair of joints). These exercises are great for focusing on the development of individual muscle groups. However, the movements involved are usually not very natural and therefore not very useful outside of the gym. Popular isolation exercises include the dumbbell curl, leg extension, and calf raise.

Compound exercises involve the movement of two or more joints (or pairs of joints). These exercises are "bigger" and more difficult than isolation exercises, not only for your muscles but also for your central nervous system. They stimulate more hormone-producing tissues and maximize the release of muscle-building hormones, such as testosterone. This leads to an increase in body-wide protein synthesis and muscular development. What's more, the movements involved with compound exercises are much more natural and therefore help you to develop functional strength. Popular compound exercises include the bench press, deadlift, and barbell squat.

Unless you intend to pre-exhaust a muscle, you should always perform compound exercises before isolation exercises. The reasons are that compound exercises offer the most benefits and require the most energy, so it makes sense to give them priority. Another reason is that the isolation exercises tire individual muscles, and if these muscles are involved in the compound exercises, the compound exercises will be compromised.

Another rule related to compound and isolation exercises is that while you can lift very heavy weights with compound exercises once you have the experience, you shouldn't regularly try to lift very heavy weights with isolation exercises. The reason is that it's unwise to put too much pressure on a single joint. With compound exercises, the weight is distributed among a number of joints, making it less risky for individual joints.

Pull and push exercises

Another common exercise classification scheme is to divide them into pull and push categories. Pull exercises are those in which the target muscle contracts when the weight is pulled towards the body and lengthens when the weight is extended away from the body. Examples of pull exercises include the crunch, dumbbell curl, and lat pull-down. Push exercises are those in which the target muscle contracts when the weight is pushed away from the body and lengthens when the weight is returned towards the body. Examples of push exercises include the overhead press, bench press, and leg extension.

Primary, assistance, and auxiliary exercises

Another way in which to classify exercises is to divide them into:

- Primary
- Assistance
- Auxiliary

These categories were originally used by competitors of powerlifting and weightlifting, but have since been adopted by many bodybuilders. Powerlifting and weightlifting are the two most popular strength sports. In both sports, the competitive goal is to make the heaviest lift. Powerlifters compete for the heaviest squat, deadlift, and bench press, whereas weightlifters compete for the heaviest snatch, and clean and jerk.

The moves for which these lifters train — the squat, deadlift, clean and jerk, etc. — are known as primary moves. The lifters train for these moves by not only practicing the moves themselves but also using assistance and auxiliary exercises. Assistance and auxiliary exercises help the lifters to improve their primary moves — hence "assistance" and "auxiliary".

Assistance exercises are usually similar to the primary move, but less intense, often dropping the barbell and replacing it either with dumbbells or body weight. For example, the dumbbell bench press and push-up are assistance exercises for the barbell bench press. Auxiliary exercises, on the other hand, are not similar to the primary move. They are usually isolation exercises that help to strengthen lagging body parts that are important for the primary move. For example, any exercise used to strengthen the shoulders to improve the clean and jerk can be considered an auxiliary exercise.

Many bodybuilders now use these terms to describe the exercises that they perform. They classify the most important exercises in their program (usually the compound exercises, such as the barbell squat, bench press, deadlift, and overhead press) as primary exercises, and they classify any exercises that help to improve these exercises as either assistance or auxiliary depending on how they assist. This, then, means that whether an exercise is primary, assistance, or auxiliary is relative to the bodybuilder's training program. Note, however, that primary and assistance exercises are almost always compound exercises, whereas auxiliary exercises are almost always isolation exercises.

When training, primary, accessory, and auxiliary exercises have to be completed in the right order. Since the primary exercises are the most important and require the most energy, they should be performed first. The accessory exercises should come next, followed by the auxiliary exercises, the latter of which will put the finishing touches to the workout.

I should also point out that some bodybuilders do not distinguish between assistance and auxiliary exercises, simply labeling them both as either assistance or auxiliary.

Aerobic and anaerobic exercises

You may also have heard of aerobic and anaerobic exercises, which I briefly explain below. For a far more detailed explanation of aerobic and anaerobic training, see the **Basics of exercise physiology** in the **Cardio Guide**.

Your body is made of cells. The cells need energy to work. They get the energy by breaking down nutrients. In order to break the nutrients down, they can either use oxygen or other chemicals. The process of using oxygen is slow but very efficient, releasing a lot of energy. The process of using the other chemicals is fast but very inefficient, producing far less energy.

When you perform low-intensity exercises, such as jogging, your cells are able to rely on the slow but efficient method of breaking nutrients down using oxygen. These exercises are known as aerobic, which means "with oxygen". However, when you perform high-intensity exercises, such as sprinting, your cells must rely on the fast but inefficient method of breaking nutrients down using the other chemicals. These exercises are known as anaerobic, which means "without oxygen".

During anaerobic exercises, muscle cells produce waste materials that lead to discomfort and weakening of the muscles. This deterioration in performance is known as **fatigue**. Fatigue forces you to lower the intensity of the activity and eventually stop, which allows the muscles to remove the waste materials. Aerobic exercises do not produce the same waste materials, which is why the muscle cells can contract repeatedly for long periods of time without fatigue.

Basically, whether an exercise is aerobic or anaerobic depends on the intensity at which you perform it. The more intensely you engage the exercise, the more anaerobic it will become. Unless you use extremely light weights, all weight training exercises are anaerobic because the muscle cells need a rapid source of energy to sustain their work.

How many sets and reps should you do?

When you train, for each exercise, you have to perform a certain number of sets and reps, and lift a specific amount of weight. The question then follows, how do you decide how many sets and reps to do for each exercise, and how much weight to lift in each set?

Muscle properties

The number of sets and reps you do, and the amount of weight that you lift, depend on what muscle property you are trying to develop. Muscles have four properties:

1. Strength (the amount of force a muscle can produce)
2. Size (a muscle's diameter)
3. Endurance (a muscle's ability to keep contracting against resistance)
4. Power (a muscle's ability to produce both strength and speed)

How to develop each property

In order to develop each property, you have to perform a different number of sets and reps. You also have to lift a different amount of weight. The following guidelines, summarized in Table 3.1, provide a generalized outline of how each muscle property can be developed.

	Strength	Power	Size	Endurance
Sets per exercise	2–6	3–5	3–6	2–3
Reps per set	2–6 (low)	1–5 (low)	6–12 (moderate)	>12 (high)
Weight (% 1RM)	Very heavy (>85)	Heavy (75–90)	Heavy (67–85)	Low–Moderate (<67)
Rest between sets	2–5 min	2–5 min	30–90 s	<30 s
Training tempo*	1:2:2	Explosive:1	2:2:3	2:2:3

Table 3.1. Guidelines for developing different muscle properties. 1RM = one-repetition maximum; min = minutes; s = seconds. *Training tempo defines the number of counts for the concentric, hold, and eccentric phases of the rep; e.g. 1:2:2 is 1 count concentric, 2 counts hold, and 2 counts eccentric.

What is 1RM?

Notice that the amount of weight you have to lift to develop each property is presented relative to your **1RM**, which stands for **one-repetition maximum** (or one-rep max for short). Your 1RM is the heaviest weight that you can lift in an exercise for one, and only one, rep using proper form. Being aware of your 1RM for a given exercise can be useful for two reasons:

1. You can use it to work out how much weight to lift for the exercise (although this isn't necessary, as explained below).
2. It allows you to notice and measure an increase in strength. If your 1RM increases, you know that you have become stronger. If it doesn't increase, it means that you have hit a **plateau**.

You can find your 1RM for a given exercise by working up to it using increasingly heavier weights, or by estimating it by finding a weight with which you can perform three reps (which is safer) and consulting a 1RM chart. By convention, the weight with which you can perform one rep is known as your 1RM, the weight with which you can perform two reps is called your 2RM, and so on.

Note, however, that you don't have to know your 1RM for an exercise in order to determine the amount of weight you have to lift for that exercise. The rep range you have to follow actually tells you the amount of weight you have to lift. For example, the rep range to develop size is six to 12 reps. This means that you have to use a weight with which you can squeeze six to 12 clean reps. If you can't do six clean reps, it's too heavy; if you can easily do 12 clean reps, it's too light. In other words, by the sixth or twelfth rep, you should be nearing failure to perform clean reps. By "clean", I of course mean using proper form.

How do you develop muscular strength?

As you can see from Table 3.1, training for strength involves performing two to six sets per exercise, each consisting of two to six reps, using very heavy weights (more than 85% of your 1RM). Because the weights are very heavy, the rest interval between sets is relatively long (two to five minutes) to allow for sufficient recovery. Lifting very heavy weights ensures that virtually all Type I, Type IIa, and Type IIb muscle fibers are recruited. However, mostly muscular strength and size are developed; muscular endurance is not developed due to the small number of reps. What's more, the gains in size that you make with this rep range are not optimal. (Muscle fiber types and their properties were covered in Chapter 2, in **Muscle structure** and **How muscles work**.)

How do you develop muscular size?

Training for optimal size involves performing three to six sets, each consisting of six to 12 reps, using heavy weights (67%–85% of your 1RM). This kind of training will recruit most Type I, Type IIa, and Type IIb muscle fibers, leading to great gains in strength and size but limited gains in endurance due again to the relatively small number of reps. More size is built than with training for strength because the muscle sustains more microdamage as a result of the higher workload and the extra time under tension. This kind of training is also more effective at increasing the body's production of testosterone and growth hormone, which are important for building muscle.

How do you develop muscular endurance?

Training for endurance involves performing two to three sets, each consisting of 13 or more reps (often 15 to 20), using low to moderate weights (less than 67% of your 1RM). This kind of training will mostly recruit

Type I muscle fibers, thus helping you to develop good endurance but limited size and strength. Because the rest interval is short and the number of reps is high, sets are kept to a maximum of three to avoid overtraining.

How do you develop muscular size, strength, and endurance?

If you perform a mixture of low-rep training with heavy weights and high-rep training with moderate weights, you will recruit and strengthen the properties of all muscle fiber types and therefore develop good size, strength, and endurance.

How do you develop muscular power?

Power is developed by rapidly performing one to five reps using a heavy weight (75% to 90% of your 1RM), which recruits all fiber types but calls mainly on the properties of Type IIb muscle fibers. If performing just one or two reps, use 80% to 90% of your 1RM; if performing three to five reps, use 75% to 85% of your 1RM. The number of sets is kept between three and five, with a two- to five-minute rest between sets. Power-building exercises involve generating a great force as rapidly as possible. Such exercises can be dangerous for beginners, so they are only recommended for intermediate and advanced lifters. To avoid injury, the exercises must be performed using optimal form, after fully warming up.

Differences between small and large muscle groups

I should make it clear at this point that small muscle groups need fewer sets than do large muscle groups. Therefore, stick to the lower end of the set range for small muscle groups and the higher end of the set range for large muscle groups. What's more, small muscle groups don't require as much weight. Therefore, stick to the higher end of the rep range (and therefore the lower amount of weight) for small muscle groups and the lower end of the rep range (and therefore the higher amount of weight) for large muscle groups.

The reason that you shouldn't go too heavy on small muscle groups is that they are usually trained using isolation exercises, which, by definition, involve a single joint, and you don't want to put too much pressure on the joint. It's less risky to go heavy with compound exercises, which, of course, involve more than one joint. What's more, the heavier the weight, the more the surrounding muscle groups will get involved in the exercise, so the goal of isolating the muscle will be defeated.

Basic methods of training

As you're aware, sets and reps represent the basic building blocks of weight training. Let's now look at some of the different types of set. We'll start with the most basic and common types, before exploring the more advanced types.

Straight sets

A typical training program designed for muscular growth (hypertrophy) might ask that you perform, for example, three sets of 10 reps for the bench press, thus:

- Set 1: 10 reps
- Set 2: 10 reps
- Set 3: 10 reps

(Remember that the amount of weight you have to lift is expressed in the number of reps you have to complete. For example, a training program that asks you to complete 10 reps is asking you to use a weight with which performing 10 clean reps is challenging. If you can't do 10 clean reps, the weight is too heavy; if you can easily do 10 clean reps, it's too light.)

These types of sets are known as **straight sets** because the number of reps and the amount of weight being lifted remain the same in each set. Straight sets can also have a rep range:

- Set 1: 8–12 reps
- Set 2: 8–12 reps
- Set 3: 8–12 reps

The rep range not only allows for daily fluctuations of ability but also the natural reduction in the number of reps that you can perform with each set.

Pyramid sets

Straight sets represent the basic method of training and work perfectly well, but you will also often encounter **pyramid sets** in training programs. In a pyramid set sequence, you reduce the number of reps and increase the weight:

- Set 1: 12 reps
- Set 2: 9 reps
- Set 3: 6 reps

Note that the first set should not be easy. For each and every set, you must choose an amount of weight that makes the set challenging and pushes you to near failure. The purpose of the pyramid sequence is not to warm up the muscle group and prepare it for the heaviest set at the end; you should have already warmed up before starting the sequence.

The pyramid set sequence is probably the most popular among experienced gym-goers. It has been extensively tried and tested, and has proven to work well for numerous professional bodybuilders. However, some argue that it is not optimal and that you can get better results with straight sets or **reverse pyramid sets** (explained below). One of the reasons is that when trying to build muscle (or curves if you're a lady), your goal is to gradually increase the amount of weight that you lift, and pyramid training makes this difficult by draining your muscles before you get to the heaviest set.

Reverse pyramid sets

The reverse pyramid sequence is the pyramid sequence in reverse:

- Set 1: 6 reps
- Set 2: 9 reps
- Set 3: 12 reps

This sequence can be dangerous for beginners and should only be attempted after a thorough warmup.

Advocates of the reverse pyramid sequence say that it's better than pyramid training because it's more intense and allows you to tackle the heaviest weight when you're fresh. It also allows you to better gauge an increase in your strength, which will be an indication that you can progress to a heavier weight.

Training to failure

Mention should also be made at this point of **training to failure**, which is a very common **intensity training technique**. It involves performing reps until you can no longer complete the concentric phase of the movement using proper form. A training program may ask that in some sets you should train to failure instead of completing a certain number of reps, thus:

- Set 1: 8 reps
- Set 2: 8 reps
- Set 3: Until failure

Some training programs may even ask that you train past failure by using **assisted reps** or **dropsets**, which we'll look at soon.

Whether training to failure is beneficial or detrimental is hotly debated. On the one side you have people who say that "Training to failure is training to fail", while on the other side you have people who urge you to squeeze out every last rep, such as when Arnold Schwarzenegger famously said: "The last three or four reps is what makes the muscle grow."

Those who are against training to failure point out that it can dramatically drain your muscle cells of energy, increase resting levels of the catabolic hormone cortisol, and suppress anabolic growth factors, such as insulin-like growth factor 1 (IGF-1) — all of which can hinder long-term growth. On the other hand, those who support training to failure point out that it ensures greater metabolic stimulation, more Type II muscle fiber recruitment, and an increased production of lactic acid in the muscles, which is important for muscle growth because it triggers an increase in intramuscular growth factors.

The question therefore follows, is training to failure good or bad? Most now agree that it should be used, but sparingly, in which case it can be beneficial. Training to failure should only be used on the last set or two of a given exercise, and shouldn't be used in every workout. Alternating the strategy on a weekly basis is often recommended. Note, however, that training to failure makes proper nutrition and adequate rest even more important.

Advanced methods of training

Now that we have looked at the basic methods of training, let's explore some of the more advanced methods, such as assisted training, dropset training, rest–pause training, eccentric training, compound and superset training, and pre-exhaustion training. These types of training (also known as **intensity training techniques**) become increasingly important as you gain training experience and start to notice that making gains has become more difficult.

Assisted training

The concept of assisted training is very simple. It basically involves getting a spotter or training partner to help you to do a few more reps after the point of failure. The extra reps will help to increase muscle overload.

It's important that your spotter doesn't help you too much. He or she should only assist you in keeping the weight moving through the sticking point. Any more help than that and you will not get much benefit from doing the extra reps.

Since assisted reps are even more demanding than training to failure, they are controversial. If you want to try assisted reps, limit them to the last set of a given exercise, and don't use them every week.

Dropset training

Dropsets are another way of training past failure, this time without the need for a spotter or training partner. As with assisted reps, the concept is simple: After you hit failure, just continue the exercise with a lighter weight, without resting. Then, after you hit failure again, you can continue with an even lighter weight. Since you'll be dropping the amount of weight each time, you'll start by stimulating Type II fibers in the heavy set, and then stimulate Type I fibers as the weight gets lighter, thus allowing you to train for strength, size, and endurance within the same set.

Dropsets are obviously suited for dumbbell and machine exercises, which allow you to change the weight quickly and safely. As with assisted reps, limit the technique to the last set of a given exercise, and don't use it every week.

Rest–pause training

Rest–pause training is as simple a concept as assisted and dropset training: Once you hit failure, put down the weights, wait for 15 to 20 seconds, pick the weights back up, and continue until failure again. To give your muscles a chance to recover, limit the technique to the last set of a given exercise, and don't use it every week.

Compound and superset training

Compound and superset training involve performing two sets in a row without resting. If the sets target the same muscle group, it's known as a **compound set**; if the sets target different or opposing muscle groups, it's known as a **superset**.

When you perform a compound set, not only is the muscle group subjected to more stress but it is also worked from different angles, thus often stimulating more muscle fibers. One example would be to perform the dumbbell fly immediately after the barbell bench press. As you can imagine, this kind of set sequence is very demanding and should therefore be used sparingly.

Note that if you perform more than two sets in a row that target the same muscle group, it's known as a **giant set**.

Supersets are less demanding than compound sets. One example of a superset in which opposing muscle groups are trained is to perform a set of dumbbell curls followed by a set of triceps extensions. Superset training is beneficial for three reasons:

1. Since there is no resting time between the sets, the workout time is reduced.
2. The intensity of the workout is increased.
3. The lack of a resting period between the sets and the resultant increase in intensity provides a better cardiovascular workout.

Eccentric training

Eccentric training (also known as **negative training**) involves doing sets using extremely heavy weights that you are unable to lift by yourself (up to 140% of your 1RM). Spotters assist you in completing the concentric phases of the reps, but allow you to complete the eccentric phases by yourself, very slowly and carefully. The reasoning behind this method of training is that, as explained in **Guidelines and principles**, eccentric phases of reps have more muscle-splitting potential than do concentric phases, which means that eccentric training could lead to greater muscle growth.

Eccentric training should be reserved for advanced lifters. It can be very dangerous, and causes greater muscle soreness than usual due to greater muscle fiber damage. Advanced lifters may sometimes perform entire workouts using just negative training, sometimes to help them break out of a plateau. Because of the increased amount of microdamage to muscles, sets are limited to just three or four per muscle group, the resting time between sets is increased, and up to two weeks are allowed before performing another eccentric workout (concentric workouts are performed in between as normal, after a few days' rest). Eccentric sets can also be used during a regular workout, in which case they should be limited to the last set of a given exercise, and they should not be used every week.

Pre-exhaustion training

Pre-exhaustion training, also known as **pre-tiring** or **pre-fatiguing** training, involves partially exhausting the prime mover muscle(s) of a certain body part by performing an isolation exercise before moving on to a compound exercise. Sometimes, two isolation exercises are performed before the compound exercise, in which case it is known as a **double pre-exhaustion**. One example is to pre-exhaust the quadriceps with a set or two of leg extensions before performing the barbell squat. Another example is to pre-exhaust the glutes with a set or two of standing cable hip extensions before performing the barbell deadlift.

Pre-exhaustion training can be used for different reasons. For example, a pain in your knee might limit the number of squats you can do, so you might pre-exhaust your quadriceps before doing squats to ensure that your quadriceps get a thorough workout. However, the most common reason for pre-exhausting prime movers is to ensure that they work twice as hard on compound exercises, which can help you to get a better workout or even break through a plateau. Another reason for pre-exhaustion training is simply to enjoy a change in your workout.

Safety always comes first

Training can be dangerous. Your main focus when working out should not be to develop your muscles but rather to stay safe and injury free. If you hurt yourself, you could take yourself out of the gym for months, during which time you will lose a lot, or even all, of your gains. You could even hurt yourself permanently. Although serious injuries are rare, they are a genuine threat, so it's important to keep gym safety in mind. Worse still, if you do not follow gym safety guidelines, you could hurt someone else.

Below I have provided a list of tips that will help you to stay safe in the gym. Although they are quite straightforward, you'll be surprised at how often even experienced gym-goers tend to forego simple gym safety guidelines, thus risking their safety and the safety of other gym-goers. Try not to make the same mistake.

Gym safety tips

Wear appropriate clothing

Keep clothes tucked in and shoelaces tied. Don't wear overly loose or tight clothing. Loose clothing can get snagged, and tight clothing can restrict your movement, which can hinder your balance, as well as prevent you from achieving a full range of motion.

Warm up before you train

Warming up will prepare your mind and body for exercise, which can prevent a variety of possible injuries. Warming up is covered in detail in the next chapter, in **How to warm up**.

Lock your plates

Locking your weight plates every time can be tedious, but it's far safer than training with loose plates. If you break form or lose balance, the loose plates can obviously fall off — hopefully, not onto someone else!

Check barbell sleeves

A loaded Olympic barbell includes the barbell, the thick sleeves that are screwed onto the bar at each end, the weight plates that are slotted onto the sleeves, and the collars that keep the plates from falling off. Note that the sleeves themselves can become loose and fall off, complete with the plates and collars. Therefore, always check that the nuts of the sleeves are secure before using a barbell.

Dismount heavy bars carefully

On at least three occasions I have loaded a very heavy bar, snatched it off the rack too aggressively, and nearly lost balance. Once, the bar nearly came crashing down onto my legs while lying on a bench! With that in mind, dismount heavy bars slowly and carefully.

Use a belt when you lift very heavy

A high-quality weightlifting belt may help to prevent lower back injuries, as well as provide support for your core muscles, when you lift very heavy. However, use the belt only when you lift very heavy, otherwise you will grow dependent on it and compromise the strengthening of your lower back and core muscles.

Practice proper form

Proper form doesn't just ensure that you get maximum results but also reduces the risk of injury. Always have complete control over the weight.

Follow the correct breathing pattern

When you perform heavy compound exercises, many of your muscles get involved, all of which require oxygen. They leach the oxygen out of your bloodstream, momentarily leaving little oxygen for your brain. If you hold your breath or fail to breathe adequately while exerting yourself, the lack of oxygen going to your brain can cause you to faint. Therefore, be mindful of your breathing pattern. As a general rule, you should exhale while performing the concentric phase of a rep and inhale while performing the eccentric phase.

Don't go too heavy

It can be tempting for guys to show off in front of their gym buddies and use weights that are overly heavy — especially if their buddies lift heavy weights. Do not be one of these individuals. All you will be doing is compromising proper form, placing unnecessary stress on your bones, joints, ligaments, and tendons, and risking an injury.

Train with a partner or spotter

When you lift heavy weights, always get someone to spot you. A spotter is someone who guides and guards you while you're lifting. Ideally, your spotter should be someone who could actually stop a barbell from hurting you. If you don't have a training partner, ask a gym-goer to spot you. Most gym-goers have a fraternal attitude, and spotting each other is normal. Even if your spotter can't stop the accident from happening, he or she can still call for help if an accident occurs.

Use a power rack

In the absence of a spotter, use a power rack (aka power cage). A power rack will allow you to train alone safely. It is basically a metal frame with adjustable safety bars that can prevent heavy barbells from flattening your person. For example, if you want to bench press in a power rack, just place the bench inside and set the safety bars above your chest. You will then not have to worry about the bar flattening your chest if you can't press it up. It's the same for barbell squats. Just position the safety bars a little below the height to which you want to squat. If you fail to complete a squat, just fall forward and crawl out.

Rerack your plates

Try not to be one of the inconsiderate individuals who leaves plates and dumbbells lying all over the floor. When you've finished with your equipment, place it back in its proper place. This not only promotes the safety of gym-goers but also keeps the gym tidy and makes equipment easier to find.

Be aware of your surroundings

Not everyone in the gym is as mindful as you are. Keep your eyes open for risks posed by other gym-goers, many of whom do not follow even the most basic gym safety guidelines.

Learn about your body and your exercises

Knowledge and understanding of the biomechanics of your body and the movement patterns of the exercises can help you to avoid injuries, as well as practice the best possible form and get the most out of your workouts. The more you know about your body and the exercises that you perform, the less likely you will be to hurt yourself.

Avoid dangerous exercises

Steer clear of exercises that are known to be dangerous, such as:

- dumbbell fly
- upright row
- behind-the-neck lat pull-down
- behind-the-neck pull-up
- behind-the-neck press.

The first two exercises (the dumbbell fly and upright row) are only dangerous if you do them incorrectly, whereas the remaining behind-the-neck exercises should be avoided at all costs.

Chapter 4: Getting started and succeeding

How to get started with weight training

Define your goals

One of the most important things you can do before setting off on any mission is to clearly define your end goal. Why do you want to train? Is it to lose weight? Build muscle? Improve your figure? Enhance your sporting performance? If so, your goal is *not* clear enough.

For the best possible chance of achieving your goal, your goal must be SMART:

1. Specific
2. Measurable
3. Agreed
4. Realistic
5. Time-bound

Specific

Being very specific about your long-term goal will help you to focus on the task at hand and stay on track. Think carefully about exactly what you want to achieve through training and write it down. For example, "I want to lose 15 pounds of fat and add 20 pounds of muscle in one year" might be a decent goal for a guy, whereas "I want to lose 15 pounds of fat and add 10 pounds of muscle in one year" might be a decent goal for a lady. In fact, it would be better to be even more specific and write down the exact body measurements (biceps, chest, waist, glutes, body-fat percentage, etc.) you wish to attain. You could also write down how much weight you wish to be able to lift with key exercises, such as the bench press, deadlift, and squat.

In addition to having specific long-term (yearly) goals, you should have specific short-term (monthly or quarterly) goals. The short-term goals should be designed to drive you towards your long-term goals. For example, if you want to add 20 pounds of muscle in one year, you will have to add five pounds each quarter.

Measurable

Your long-term and short-term goals should be measurable and trackable. The examples I gave of defining a specific amount of fat you want to lose, muscle you want to gain, weight you want to lift, or body measurement you want to achieve are ideal. If you can't measure and track your progress, you will not know whether or not you are making the right kinds of gains and therefore nearing your short-term and long-term goals. For guidance, see **How to track your progress**, later in this chapter.

Agreed

To increase your likelihood of sticking to your short-term and long-term goals, discuss and agree upon your goals with your fitness instructor, training partner, or friend. Commit the goals to paper in the form of mission statements, sign and date it, and get the other party to sign it as a witness. Place the "contract" somewhere where you can always see it so that it can remind you of your goals. Taking this extra measure will promote more commitment and focus to achieving your goals.

Realistic

Your short-term and long-term goals must be realistic. Be realistic about what you can actually attain in the specified amount of time, taking into account your body type, genetics, and lifestyle. Acknowledge that progress is slow and difficult, and that you will not achieve your ideal body and state of fitness any time soon. If your goals are unrealistic, you will likely fail to achieve them, in which case you will be more likely to lose motivation and give up.

Time-bound

To keep you focused and to prompt action, make sure that your short-term and long-term goals have deadlines. Without clear deadlines, you will likely procrastinate and put things off.

Choose a weight training program

Once you have decided on your SMART goals, you can choose a weight training program that will help you to achieve them. The training programs that I have provided are designed to be as effective and manageable as possible.

Decide on where you're going to train

Now that you've defined your goals and chosen your training program, you have to decide where you're going to train. You can train either at home or at a gym. The following questions will help you to decide:

- How much money do you have to spend?
- Can you afford the equipment necessary to build a decent and safe home gym?
- How good are you at motivating yourself?
- How far are you prepared to travel to a gym?
- Would you prefer to train with other people or by yourself?

If undecided, I would always recommend that you join a gym. The advantages are much more important than the disadvantages (see below). However, if possible, you should also buy essential pieces of equipment for your home (see **Set up your home gym** below). The home equipment is only for when you can't make it to the gym. It ensures that you never have an excuse not to train.

Advantages of joining a gym

- Motivational gym atmosphere

- A diverse range of equipment
- Instructors on hand to offer assistance and advice
- Fellow gym-goers with whom to make friends, train, and keep motivated
- Spotters on hand to keep you safe
- Possible access to additional facilities, such as classes, a store, swimming pool, and sauna
- Once you pay, you'll be more likely to train

Disadvantages of joining a gym

- Membership fees can sometimes be expensive
- Possible overcrowding during peak times (usually in the evening, after work, and in the morning, before work)
- May have to travel far

Advantages of training at home

- No membership fees
- Train in privacy
- No overcrowding
- Train whenever you like
- No need to travel

Disadvantages of training at home

- Essential equipment can be expensive
- Probably have a very small variety of equipment
- Likely lack big machines and cardiovascular equipment
- Less motivating environment
- No gym buddies with whom to bond and train
- No spotters for help and safety
- No instructors for advice and assistance
- Greater risk of injury
- No amenities, such as fitness classes, swimming pool, etc.

Set up your home gym

If you do decide to train at home, whether male or female, you will need the following equipment:

- An adjustable bench
- A set of dumbbells
- A barbell
- A power rack/cage for safety
- A pull-up bar
- A multipurpose cable machine OR a set of clip resistance bands
- Ankle straps

Note that power racks often feature pull-up bars, and clip resistance band packages often include ankle straps.

The equipment listed above will ensure that you can train safely and effectively, and get the most out of the weight training programs in this book. The last two items in the list are not absolutely essential because I have provided alternative exercises for all cable and machine exercises. However, they are essential if you want to perform the most effective exercises and get the best possible results, as well as dramatically increase the number of exercises that you can perform. Luckily, the set of clip resistance bands can be used to perform the equivalents of cable machine exercises, thus saving you from having to buy a multipurpose cable machine.

Clip resistance bands have come a long way. Stronger than ever, they can be stacked onto handles to dramatically increase resistance. They come with door anchors and ankle straps, allowing you to perform a huge range of exercises. Being lightweight, you can also take them on your travels, where they can help you to keep making progress.

If you decide to invest in a set of stackable clip resistance bands, make sure that you buy one with proper anti-snap technology. Watch out for anti-snap technology forgeries.

Other equipment that you will need to effectively complete the exercises in the training programs include:

- an ab wheel
- dip bars (to attach to your power rack)
- a stability ball.

However, these are completely optional.

Tips for creating a great home gym

Here are some additional tips that will help you to create the kind of home gym that will serve you well and make you proud.

- Designate a spacious area for your gym. Basements and garages work well. The area must be ventilated, though.
- Lay rubber mats on the floor to prevent damage from weights.
- Hang mirrors on the walls. These will help you to observe your form, technique, and progress.
- Set up a sound system so that you can listen to music as you train.
- Hang inspiring pictures on the walls.
- Pin pictures of your progress to a pin board for motivation.

Find the right gym

If you decide to join a gym, here are some tips to help you find one that will meet your needs:

- Make sure that the gym is closer than a 15-minute drive. The farther away it is, the less likely you will be to attend regularly.
- The gym should have a wide range of equipment. There should be plenty of free weights, and multiple adjustable benches, squat racks, cable machines, weight machines, and cardiovascular machines. A couple of boxing bags are a bonus. The equipment should be high quality and well maintained, and they should be cleaned and tested regularly.
- Make sure that the gym is well ventilated and spacious, and has a motivating atmosphere.
- Try to get an idea of the kind of people who train there. Could you train with them?
- Check if the instructors are professionally qualified.
- Get the right price. Compare membership fees, taking into account any initial joining fees. Ask about deals, such as off-peak discounts. Find out if other facilities — swimming pool, etc. — are included in the price.
- Ask for a trial workout. Conduct your trial at the same time of day that you will be regularly attending so that you can see if the gym is overcrowded at that time, as well as gauge the crowd with whom you will be training.
- If you have options, try them all and see which one you prefer.

What you will need

Whether you train at home or at a gym, you will need the following essentials for every workout:

- Suitable clothing
- A towel
- A bottle of water

The towel is essential not only to wipe your sweat but also to lay it over benches that others have sweated on!

Optionally, you may need:

- an iPod/phone and headphones to listen to your own music instead of the music played at the gym
- training gloves if you don't want calluses on your hands.

And if you start lifting very heavy weights, you may also need:

- a weightlifting belt to support your lower back
- straps to improve your grip
- knee wraps to support your knees.

How to warm up

Why should you warm up?

Warming up is probably much more important than you realize. While it is important to know how to warm up properly, you should also know why you should warm up. Warming up before a workout will help you to:

- increase your body temperature
- lubricate your joints
- increase blood flow to your muscles
- loosen your muscles, joints, and connective tissues
- improve the elasticity of your muscles, enabling them to work harder, more efficiently, and for longer before they fatigue
- allow nerve impulses to be transmitted faster
- increase your mental alertness and awareness
- prepare mentally for your workout
- rehearse proper form and technique
- establish a mental connection with, and "pre-activate", the target muscle group.

All of the above will reduce your chances of sustaining an injury and increase your body's ability to work and therefore make gains. Warming up can also boost your arousal and motivation.

How to warm up properly

I recommend the following warm-up sequence:

1. Perform five to 10 minutes of dynamic stretching (explained below).
2. Do some cardio for five to 10 minutes on the treadmill, elliptical cross-trainer, rowing machine, or exercise bike. Make sure to break into a sweat.
3. Warm up the target muscle group(s) with a light set using approximately 50% of the weight that you will be using in the workout.
4. Do a heavier set using approximately 75% of the weight that you will be using in the workout.

You can then safely start your workout.

Note that the heavier the weight you will be using in the workout, the more warmup sets you will have to do to prepare your target muscles for the heavy weight. For example, if it is leg day and you have to squat 250 pounds, you should do a few squats each using, for example, 150 pounds, 175 pounds, 200 pounds, and 225 pounds. On the other hand, if you will not be lifting very heavy weights, two lighter sets, as described above, should be more than enough to get you warmed up and ready to safely start.

Must you warm up every muscle group?

Depending on your training program, you will most likely have to train different muscle groups in each workout instead of just one muscle group. For example, Monday might be back and biceps; Tuesday might be chest, shoulders, and triceps; and Wednesday might be legs and core. You may therefore be wondering whether or not you have to perform warmup exercises for each muscle group.

If you're training your back and biceps, you only need a single compound pulling exercise (for example, the seated cable row) to warm up all of the day's target muscles. The reason is that compound pulling exercises involve your back, posterior shoulders, and elbow flexors (biceps brachii, brachialis, and brachioradialis). Indeed, this is also the very reason that people often train back and biceps together. Similarly, if you're training your chest, shoulders, and triceps, you only need a single compound pushing exercise (for example, the push-up) to warm up all of the day's target muscles. The reason is that compound pushing exercises involve your chest, anterior shoulders, and triceps.

If you're training muscle groups that do not work together, such as opposing muscle groups (for example, chest and back), then you will need a warmup exercise for each one.

Pre-activation movements

Having a strong mind–muscle connection as you train is believed to help recruit more muscle fibers, leading to greater gains. Therefore, you should always be focusing on your muscles and the movement patterns as you train, and you should strive to establish the connection in the warmup. The compound warmup exercises will usually suffice to make the connection; however, some people find making the connection with certain muscles difficult, in which case they employ **pre-activation movements** for assistance. Pre-activation movements can be compound or isolation exercises — basically, any exercise that helps the individual to make the mind–muscle connection. For example, to activate the glutes, ladies might use single-leg hip thrusts or various loop band exercises, whereas to activate the lats, men might use single-arm lat pull-downs.

What is dynamic stretching?

The warmup procedure I recommended above starts with five to 10 minutes of **dynamic stretching**. Dynamic stretching is different from the type of stretching with which you are probably familiar, known as **static stretching**. Static stretching involves holding a position for 30 or so seconds in order to elongate the muscle. Dynamic stretching, on the other hand, is a newer variation of stretching that involves performing fluid, controlled movements that take your joints safely through their full range of motion without stretching the muscles.

Unfortunately, I can't describe the actual stretches here. Please see the video at the bottom of the following page of my website for a demonstration:

http://weighttraining.guide/training/how-to-warm-up/

You should perform dynamic stretching and not static stretching as part of your warmup sequence because the latter can impede the performance of your muscles, as well as lead to an injury when done before your muscles and joints are warmed up. Note, however, that static stretching is recommended *after* your workout, during your cooldown.

How to cool down

Post-workout static stretching

Many individuals understand the importance of the warmup before the workout but fail to appreciate the importance of the cooldown. Indeed, most people aren't even aware that such a thing exists, let alone know how to cool down properly.

The cooldown is very straightforward. It basically involves gently stretching the muscles that you trained during your workout, and only takes five to 10 minutes. The type of stretching that you do is static stretching as opposed to the dynamic stretching that you did as part of your warmup.

Benefits of static stretching

As explained above, static stretching is the regular kind of stretching that involves holding a position for approximately 30 seconds in order to elongate the muscle. Although static stretching is not suitable as part of your warmup, it can be beneficial after your workout because it can help to prevent a reduction in the range of motion of your joints, which may occur if you consistently perform reps with a partial range of motion. But that's not all. Static stretching, whether performed after a workout or by itself, can also help to:

- improve your flexibility by increasing the range of motion of your joints and stretching your muscles, tendons, ligaments, and skin
- keep your muscle tissues, tendons, and ligaments strong, which reduces your risk of sustaining injuries, such as straining a muscle or tearing a tendon
- reduce your chances of developing problems associated with muscle tightness, such as joint instability
- improve your posture, mobility, and gait
- make room for muscle growth by elongating the connective tissue (fascia) that covers your muscles
- relieve tension that has built up in your muscles, helping you to relax
- improve your awareness of your body and its limitations regarding movement and flexibility.

Note that static stretching has no significant effect on preventing or reducing muscle soreness, which is now considered to be a myth.

The science of static stretching

In order to stretch properly and effectively, a very basic understanding of the science of stretching is necessary. In particular, you need to be aware of the two protective muscle reflexes. The reason is that in order to stretch properly, you will have to work around one of the reflexes and work with the other reflex. The two protective reflexes are called the **stretch reflex** and **autogenic inhibition**.

What is the stretch reflex?

Each of your skeletal muscles contains receptors called **muscle spindles**, which monitor changes in the length of the muscle and the rate at which the change in length occurs. If the muscle is rapidly stretched, the muscle spindles initiate a reflex that makes the muscle contract. This is the stretch reflex, and its purpose is to stop the muscle from overstretching and getting damaged.

What is autogenic inhibition?

Unlike the stretch reflex, which forces your muscles to contract, autogenic inhibition forces your muscles to relax. This reflex is initiated by receptors called **Golgi tendon organs (GTOs)**, which are located in your tendons (the connective tissues that attach your muscles to your bones). GTOs monitor the amount of tension that builds up in your tendons during muscle contractions. If the tension is excessive, GTOs cause the associated muscles to relax, thus reducing or eliminating the tension and preventing damage to muscles and tendons caused by excessive forces.

How to stretch properly

In order to effectively stretch a muscle, you have to avoid initiating the stretch reflex and instead initiate autogenic inhibition. You avoid the stretch reflex by easing into the stretch slowly, and you initiate autogenic inhibition by holding the stretch for longer than six seconds. This will cause the muscle to relax, lengthen, and remain in a stretched position, allowing you to stretch it a little further. If you were to stretch the muscle rapidly, the stretch reflex would be initiated, forcing the muscle to contract and preventing any significant stretch from occurring.

How stretching can help to increase your strength and power

This benefit of stretching was left out of the list of benefits above because it requires understanding of GTOs and autogenic inhibition. Put simply, stretching can help to improve your strength and power by increasing the threshold at which GTOs initiate autogenic inhibition. The higher the threshold, the more weight you will be able to lift and the more intensely you will be able to train without being inhibited by GTO activation. This, in turn, will lead to greater gains in muscular size, strength, and power. Your GTO threshold will increase as your tendons become stronger as a result of both stretching and weight training.

General stretching guidelines

- Ideally, you should stretch immediately after your workout, while your muscles and tendons are still warm. You can also stretch muscles between sets, but only if you have finished training the muscles and have moved on to training other muscles.

- If you perform static stretching sessions by themselves, separate from your workouts, make sure that you warm up first with five to 10 minutes of dynamic stretching and/or cardio.
- Avoid bouncing during the stretch, which can cause injuries and initiate the stretch reflex.
- Always ease into the stretch slowly, and keep your focus on relaxing the muscle as much as possible.
- Stretch only as far as is comfortable, and hold the position for up to 30 seconds.
- Breathe normally as you stretch.
- Release the stretch slowly.

The stretches

Kneeling hip flexor stretch

1. Take a very large step forward and gently lower your back knee to the floor. You can also kneel and then take a large step forward.
2. Place your hands on your front knee.
3. Keeping your body upright and facing forward, press your back hip forward.
4. Hold the stretch.
5. Repeat with your opposite leg.

Main muscles stretched: Iliopsoas of back leg, and Gluteus Maximus and Adductor Magnus of front leg

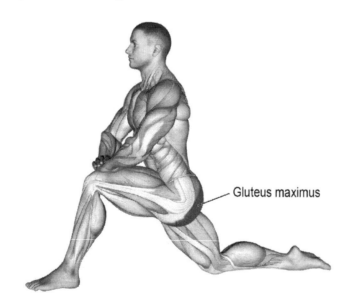

Gluteus maximus

Lying glute stretch

1. Lie on your back on the floor with your knees bent and your feet flat on the floor.
2. Cross the lower leg of one leg over the thigh of the other leg.
3. With both hands, grasp the back of the thigh upon which you rested the other leg and pull it toward your torso.
4. Hold the stretch.
5. Repeat with your opposite leg.

Main muscles stretched: Gluteus Maximus

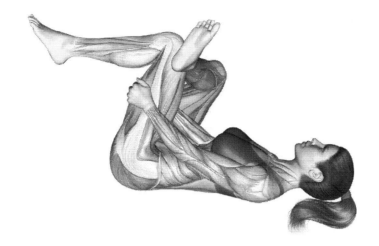

Standing quadriceps stretch

1. Hold on to a sturdy object with one hand for balance.
2. Bend your opposite leg behind you and grasp the front of your ankle.
3. Keeping your knees close together, straighten your hip by moving your knee backward.
4. Hold the stretch.
5. Repeat with your opposite leg.

Main muscles stretched: Quadriceps

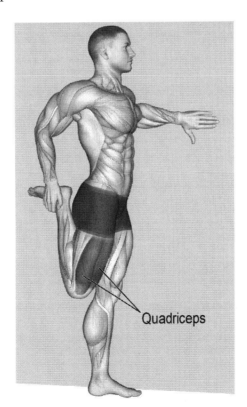

Seated hamstrings stretch

1. Sit on the floor with your legs apart and knees straight.
2. Reach forward and grasp one foot.
3. Hold the stretch.
4. Repeat with your opposite leg.

Main muscles stretched: Hamstrings, Erector Spinae

Alternatively, if it makes it easier for you, you can bend the leg that is not being stretched, as in the illustration.

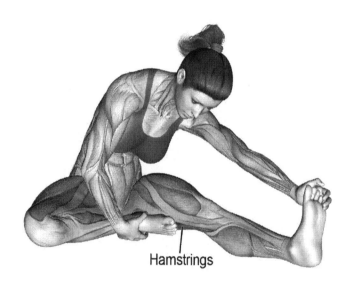

Hamstrings

Seated adductor stretch

1. Sit on the floor and bring the soles of your feet together.
2. Grasp your feet and pull them close to your body.
3. Press your thighs or lower legs downward with your elbows.
4. Hold the stretch.

Main muscles stretched: Adductor Brevis, Adductor Longus, Adductor Magnus

You do not have to keep your back straight. In fact, you can use the opportunity to stretch your lower back (erector spinae) as well. If you lean forward, you can also stretch your gluteus maximus.

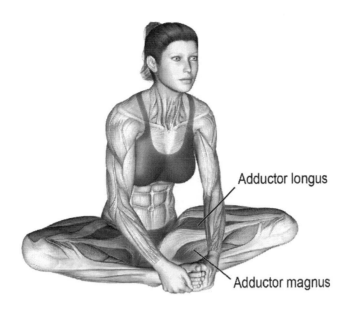

Adductor longus

Adductor magnus

Calf stretch

1. With your hands on your hips and both feet pointing forward, take a step backward with one leg and gently lower your heel to the floor.
2. Keeping both feet flat and your torso upright, straighten your back leg. Your front knee should be directly above your front foot.
3. Hold the stretch.
4. Repeat with your opposite leg.

Main muscles stretched: Gastrocnemius, Iliopsoas

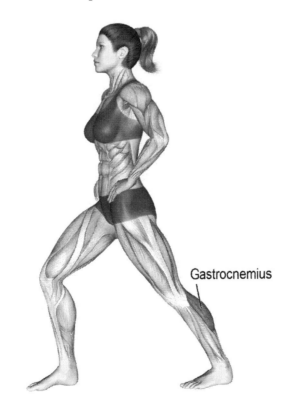

Gastrocnemius

Chest and biceps stretch

1. Stand perpendicular to a wall.
2. With your arm straight, place your palm against the wall at shoulder height.
3. Slowly turn your body away from your arm.
4. Hold the stretch.
5. Repeat with your opposite arm.

Main muscles stretched: Pectoralis Major, Pectoralis Minor, Anterior Deltoid, Biceps Brachii, Brachialis, Brachioradialis

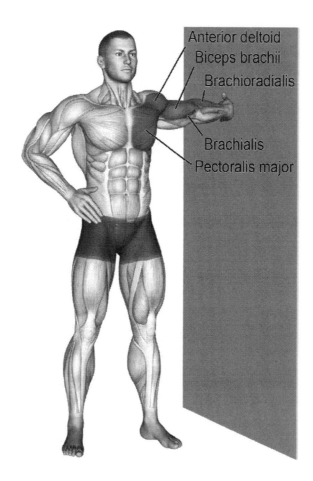

Upper back stretch

1. Stand facing something sturdy that you can hold on to, such as a bar.
2. Grasp the bar with one hand at approximately waist height.
3. Bend over and allow your hips to fall backward and your arm to stretch forward.
4. Lean into the stretched arm.
5. Hold the stretch.
6. Repeat with your opposite arm.

Main muscles stretched: Latissimus Dorsi, Teres Major, Posterior Deltoid, Lower Trapezius, Rhomboids, Infraspinatus, Teres Minor

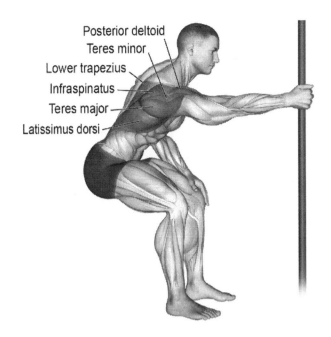

Side reach lat stretch

1. Stand with your feet spaced wide apart.
2. Place one hand on the side of your thigh and raise the other hand overhead.
3. Lean to the opposite side of your raised arm and stretch your raised arm out.
4. Hold the stretch.
5. Repeat with your opposite arm.

Main muscles stretched: Latissimus Dorsi, Teres Major

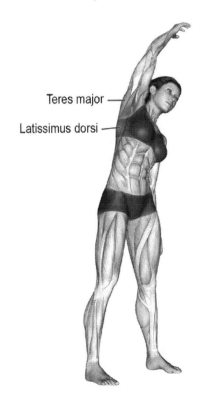

Posterior deltoid stretch

1. Place one arm across your upper chest.
2. Grasp your elbow with your other hand.
3. Push your elbow toward your upper chest.
4. Hold the stretch.
5. Repeat with your opposite arm.

Main muscles stretched: Posterior Deltoid, Infraspinatus, Teres Minor, Middle and Lower Trapezius, Rhomboids

To stretch your lateral deltoid, position your arm across your lower chest instead of across your upper chest.

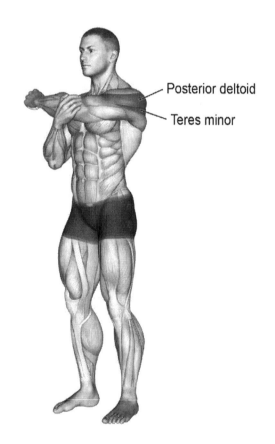

Posterior deltoid

Teres minor

Overhead triceps stretch

1. Raise one arm straight up into the air and flex your elbow as if reaching for your shoulder blades.
2. Grasp the elbow of your raised arm over your head with your other hand.
3. Pull your elbow backward.
4. Hold the stretch.
5. Repeat with your opposite arm.

Main muscles stretched: Triceps Brachii, Latissimus Dorsi, Teres Major

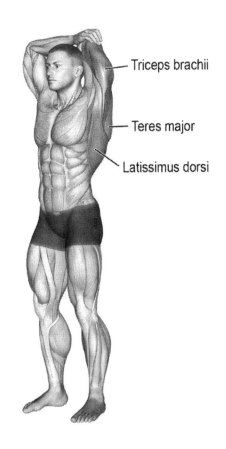

Triceps brachii

Teres major

Latissimus dorsi

Cat stretch

1. Get on your hands and knees, with your hands shoulder-width apart.
2. Flex your spine by hunching your back up.
3. Hold the stretch.

Main muscles stretched: Erector Spinae

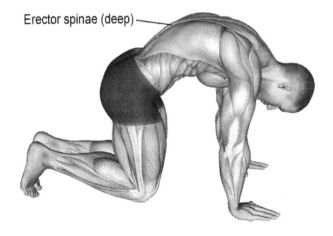

Erector spinae (deep)

Prone abdominal stretch

1. Lie prone (on your front) on the floor.
2. Place your hands on the floor to the sides of your shoulders.

3. Keeping your pelvis on the floor, push your torso up off the floor.
4. Hold the stretch.

Main muscles stretched: Rectus Abdominis, Iliopsoas

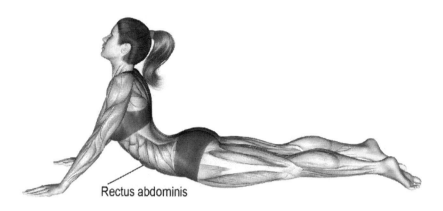

Rectus abdominis

Pretzel stretch

1. Sit on the floor with your knees straight.
2. Cross one leg over the other leg and place your foot on the floor next to your knee.
3. Twist your torso to the side of your bent leg. As you do so, you can support your body by placing your hand on the floor behind you.
4. Place the elbow of your opposite arm on the outside of your bent knee.
5. Twist your torso further by pressing your elbow against the outside of your knee.
6. Hold the stretch.
7. Repeat with your opposite side.

Main muscles stretched: Internal and External Obliques, Gluteus Medius, Gluteus Minimus, Erector Spinae

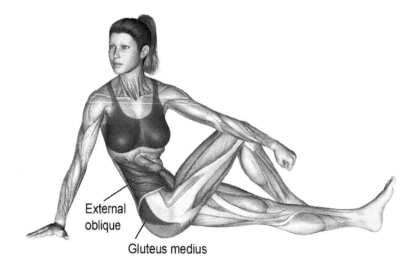

External oblique
Gluteus medius

How to track your progress

Why track your progress?

Achieving your goals will take time. Tracking your progress will let you know if your training program and diet are working. If they are, great! Keep following the same program and diet and monitoring your results. On the other hand, if they are not working, you have to take the necessary actions to get back on track.

As you track your progress, you will develop a better understanding of your body and how it responds to different stimuli. The patterns that you observe and the insights that you glean will help you to make more informed decisions and therefore assume greater control of your progress.

Monitoring your progress can also be very motivating. Looking back over your progress and seeing how far you have come can provide very strong impetus to carry on and take things further.

What should you track?

This depends on how meticulous you want to be. You can track any or all of the following:

- Body weight
- Body measurements
- Body composition, namely, your body-fat percentage

The measurements can be recorded using a measurement log or table. See Table 4.1 for an example. You should also take photos of yourself at regular intervals.

Date	Weight	Fat %	Body measurements							
			Neck	Chest	Waist	Hips	Thighs	Calves	Biceps	Forearms

Table 4.1. Progress measurement log.

How to track your body weight

To track your body weight, weigh yourself using a reliable scale every day and calculate an average every week. A weekly average is more accurate than weighing yourself once a week because your weight can fluctuate on a daily basis due to differing amounts of water retention, glycogen storage, food intake, and other factors. Weigh yourself naked every morning, before eating or drinking anything, and after going to the bathroom. Then, every seven days, add up the figures and divide the sum by seven to get your weekly average.

How to take body measurements

To take body measurements, you will need a fabric measuring tape. Measure your body parts every couple of months, in the morning, at the same time, and not after they have been exercised. Always measure the same area, usually the middle of the muscle. Don't pull the measuring tape too taut, and make sure that it's not too loose. To ensure an accurate log, always be consistent in the way that you take the measurements. Check your tape measure against a metal tape or ruler occasionally to ensure that it hasn't stretched or shrunk.

Why to track your body composition

Strictly speaking, body composition refers to the major components of your body: fat, bone, muscle, blood, etc. However, in the context of weight training and bodybuilding, it is usually used to refer to just two components:

1. Fat mass (all of the fat in your body, usually expressed as body-fat percentage)
2. Fat-free mass (everything else)

Tracking your fat mass and fat-free mass as you train and diet is important because it will help you to analyze and evaluate how your body is changing and therefore determine if you are making progress in the right direction. For example, if you are bulking (consuming an excess of calories to maximize muscle growth), you want to see your weight go up ideally due mostly to an increase in fat-free mass. This will indicate that you have added more muscle than fat. Conversely, if you are cutting (consuming fewer calories than your body needs with the aim of losing body fat), you want to see your weight go down ideally due mostly to a decrease in fat mass. This will indicate that you have lost more fat than muscle.

How to track your body-fat percentage

There are quite a few ways in which you can track your body-fat percentage, including:

- hydrostatic weighing
- bioelectric impedance analysis
- skinfold testing.

Hydrostatic weighing

The most accurate method of measuring your body-fat percentage is hydrostatic weighing (also known as **hydrodensitometry**). The method involves being weighed both outside of water and while submerged in a specialized tank of water. Your body's density is calculated by comparing the difference between the two measurements. Since fat-free mass (bone, muscle, etc.) is denser than fat mass and therefore weighs more in water, the density measurement can then be used to calculate your body-fat percentage. The problems with this method are that it is expensive (costing approximately $100 to $200) and impractical (being available only at universities and hospitals).

Bioelectric impedance analysis

Bioelectrical impedance analysis (BIA) is the technology behind the many body composition scales sold for home use. There are also hand-held devices. The technology is based on the fact that electricity flows more easily through tissues that are mostly composed of water, such as blood and muscle, than it does through tissues that have less or no water, such as bone and fat. The method involves standing barefoot on a BIA scale (or holding the handles of a BIA hand-held device), which sends a harmless electrical current through your body. The device measures the resistance (impedance) of the electrical current as it travels through your body and uses the measurement, along with other information, such as your height, weight, and gender, to predict how much body fat you have. The problem with BIA is that it's the most inaccurate of the three mentioned methods, with the results depending strongly on how hydrated you are.

Skinfold testing

Skinfold testing is probably the most common method of measuring body-fat percentage used by personal trainers. It involves using body-fat calipers to take measurements of the thickness of your skin at various sites on your body. The measurements are then summed, and the total is compared with a chart that estimates your body-fat percentage.

Body-fat calipers are cheap and usually come with clear instructions. Sometimes, the instructions request measurements to be taken from only three sites on your body; other times, measurements are requested from multiple sites. The more sites that are measured, the more accurate will be the final result. The accuracy of the final result also depends on the abilities of the individual taking the measurements (you can't take them yourself). The measurements must of course be taken properly, using a consistent method.

Note that some of the sites from which measurements are taken are different for men and women. What's more, all of the measurements are taken from one side of the body.

How to avoid overtraining

Before we can explore how to avoid overtraining and how to cure it, we must define it. There are two types of overtraining: **muscular** and **CNS**.

What is muscular overtraining?

When you train, your muscles sustain microdamage, which is normal. While you rest, your body repairs the damage and reinforces the muscles with extra proteins to protect them from future damage. That is how your muscles grow. Muscular overtraining is when you consistently train too much and fail to let your muscles recover. As a result, your muscles stop growing and you experience a plateau or a decline in training performance. You may also experience chronic (ongoing) muscle soreness, or even muscle loss!

Muscular overtraining can affect either one or all of your muscles, depending on which ones you overtrain. There is also central nervous system (CNS) overtraining, which can be more serious.

What is CNS overtraining?

Just like your muscular system, your CNS can be overworked. As it is responsible for generating all of the muscular contractions in your workouts, excessive training can exhaust it. Unlike muscular overtraining, CNS overtraining affects your entire body. General symptoms include:

- weakness and tiredness
- loss of workout motivation
- lack of enthusiasm for everyday activities
- inability to concentrate
- lack of body coordination
- inability to sleep, or difficulty waking up
- elevated heart rate while training and/or resting
- loss of appetite
- weight loss.

Who is at risk of overtraining?

You may be at risk of overtraining if you train excessively for several consecutive months, which is not recommended (see **Tips on how to avoid overtraining** below). Most people who think that they are overtraining are usually nowhere near it. Noticing that you can't do as many reps today as you could in your previous workout doesn't indicate that you have overtrained. Daily fluctuations in ability are normal. You should suspect overtraining only if you know that you have been training very intensely for many months without a break and have observed the symptoms of overtraining for multiple consecutive workouts.

How do you cure overtraining?

Fortunately, mild cases of overtraining are easy to cure: Just take a **deload week** to give your body time to recover. Basically, a deload week is a week during which you take it easy and either take some time off from training or significantly reduce the **volume** and **intensity** of your workouts. Generally speaking, volume is the number of exercises, sets, and reps that you do per muscle group in your workouts, and intensity is the amount of weight that you lift per set relative to your one-rep max.

In extreme cases of overtraining, where the individual has overtrained for several months or even years, simply taking a deload week will probably not fix the problem. Recovery from extreme cases can take many weeks or even months. If you think you might fit into this category, please seek professional advice.

Tips on how to avoid overtraining

1. Take breaks from intense training

Since both muscular and CNS overtraining are caused by an imbalance between training and recovery, the best way to prevent them is to follow a training program that allows adequate time for rest and recovery, such as any of the training programs I have provided. However, just in case you ever follow your own training program, here are some guidelines to follow:

- Do not train each muscle group (especially large muscle groups) more than two or three times a week (unless you are following a beginner's full-body training program, in which case you can train each muscle group up to four times per week).
- Allow each muscle group to rest for at least two days before hitting it again (unless you are following a beginner's full-body training program, in which case you can allow each muscle group to rest for just one day).
- Take a deload week every eight to 12 weeks.

2. Listen to your body

An important skill in preventing overtraining is being able to listen to your body. For example, if you notice that your shoulders often still feel sore when it's time to hit them again, revise your training program so that your shoulders get more time to recover.

3. Get the right amount of sleep

Sleep is essential for rest and recovery, so make sure that you get enough of it. The National Sleep Foundation recommends between seven and nine hours of sleep per day for young adults and adults. However, this applies to the general public. You may need more if you're training intensely. Listen to your body to figure out how much sleep you need.

4. Get the right nutrients

Good nutrition is essential if you want to prevent overtraining. As you're aware, your workouts will damage your muscles. Your diet must provide the raw materials necessary to repair them, as well as to build the muscles to make them stronger and less susceptible to damage. See the **Nutrition Guide** for everything you need to know about nutrition.

5. Manage your personal life

Sometimes, symptoms that indicate CNS overtraining may in fact be being caused by issues that are outside of the gym. Busy lifestyles, stressful jobs, financial issues, break-ups, and other personal problems all impact your CNS and can leave it exhausted. Therefore, if you experience what seem to be the symptoms of CNS overtraining despite having followed a balanced training program, look for possible causes in your personal life.

What is strategic overtraining?

Now that you know how to avoid overtraining, mention should also be made of **strategic overtraining** (also known as **over-reaching**). Strategic overtraining is the process of deliberately pushing yourself into a mild state of overtraining for a short period of time (two to four weeks). As a result, you experience a regression in performance. However, after you take a deload week, your performance can rebound above and beyond its previous level.

Strategic overtraining is an advanced strategy for advanced lifters and should not be attempted by beginners. It is used by advanced lifters to break out of plateaus or increase gains when making gains becomes a struggle. Beginners, who can make great gains by following a balanced training program, have absolutely no reason to practice strategic overtraining.

How to keep motivated

Developing a healthy, strong, and attractive body takes time and effort. Many guys and girls give up because they lack the discipline, patience, and motivation. More important, they lack the right mindset to succeed. Below I present the best tips I know on how to keep motivated. Use them to develop and sustain the unwavering mindset and drive necessary for long-term persistence and success.

Focus on the benefits

Weight training is one of the best possible activities you could ever take up. It's one of the most worthwhile ways in which you could spend your time. It's so good for you that as you train, you should experience a buzz and feel great about yourself. After each workout, you should feel a sense of achievement and a growing excitement that you are nearing your goal. If ever your enthusiasm wanes, just remember all of the amazing benefits that weight training has to offer, as presented in Chapter 1, in **What are the benefits of weight training?**

Visualize your success

Keep a very clear and detailed image in your mind of your ultimate goal, including how you will look and feel when you achieve it, and how people will be reacting to you when they see your amazing results. To avoid disappointment, keep your goal realistic. Visualize the experience in vivid detail, and remember that every rep gets you closer to your goal.

Create a motivating environment

If training at home, hang mirrors and inspiring pictures all over your walls. Include pictures of people you aspire to be like. Pin your mission statement/contract and photos of your progress to a pin board. Don't forget photos of yourself that you do not like, as these can be the most motivating. As you train, listen to your favorite music. Basically, do whatever you can to make your gym as inspiring and motivating as possible. Make it your special sanctum devoted to personal growth and development.

Train with a partner

Find someone who is even more devoted to health, fitness, and personal development than you are. Preferably, the individual should be ahead of you and more knowledgeable than you are so that you can learn from them. Training with a partner will help you to stay motivated, and can make your workouts much more enjoyable. You can spot each other for safety, as well as guide, challenge, and motivate each other, and push each other to perform that one extra rep.

Use a personal trainer

If you don't have a training partner but do have money to spend, get yourself a personal trainer. Personal trainers can be great at motivating you, pushing you during your workouts, and guiding you to success. They can design new training programs for you, check your form and technique, and enhance your safety. You may be able to find personal trainers at your gym. Whoever you choose, make sure that he or she is qualified and thoroughly experienced. Don't be convinced solely by their appearance.

Track your progress

Recording your progress can be very motivating. Looking back over your progress and recognizing how far you have come can provide very strong motivation to carry on and take things further. You can record and track your measurements — body weight, body-part measurements, and body composition — using measurement logs. You should also take photos of yourself at regular intervals and pin them to a board.

Join online forums

There are many people out there who are going through exactly what you're going through. They congregate in online forums, where they help and guide each other. Join a few such bodybuilding and fitness forums. Make friends. Share your goal and journey. Share your achievements, and watch how much praise you will get. Your achievements will inspire them, and their encouragement will inspire you. And of course, not only will you find lots of inspiration and motivation in online forums but you will also find lots of great information, advice, and other useful resources.

Try a different gym

If you have gym options, try a different gym for a while. The change of scenery, equipment, and atmosphere can reinvigorate your enthusiasm. You may also be able to try different exercises and make new friends.

Reward yourself

Whenever you achieve a goal or break a personal record, reward yourself with something that you enjoy, such as a trip to the movies, a meal at a nice restaurant, a night out dancing, or new clothing. The goal that you achieve doesn't have to be a big one — give yourself small rewards for minor goals (such as reaching your weekly target) and large rewards for managing significant achievements (such as your first 200-pound squat). Your achievements don't just have to relate to weight training, either; you can reward yourself for diet-related achievements as well. For example, if you manage to meet your caloric limits for a week, permit yourself a cheat meal.

PART 2: NUTRITION GUIDE

Chapter 5: Macronutrients and micronutrients

Nutrition overview

A decent understanding of nutrition is important if you want to maximize your weight training results. Along with following an effective training program and getting enough rest, adhering to an effective diet is one of the pillars of weight training success. Below I provide a general overview of nutrition, mainly as it relates to weight training. The subjects covered below will then be explored in much greater detail.

What is nutrition?

Generally speaking, **nutrition** refers to the process by which living organisms take in and utilize food materials. The same word is also used to describe food itself and the science of dietary requirements for proper health and development.

Why is nutrition important for weight training?

Nutritious food is essential for energy, metabolism, health, fitness, growth, and tissue repair. In the context of weight training, it is very important for providing adequate fuel for your workouts, and helping your body to recover and grow from exercise. Your workouts will damage your muscles. Your diet must provide the raw materials necessary to repair them, as well as build the muscles to make them stronger and less susceptible to damage.

The food that you eat will significantly affect your results. For weight training success, it is essential to understand at least the basics of nutrition. Following nutritional guidelines will help you to achieve your goals, whether they are to maximize muscle growth (hypertrophy), lose weight, maintain weight, gain weight, or minimize the storage of fat during a **bulking phase** (a period during which you consume an excess of calories to maximize muscle growth).

What do you need to know?

Gaining an understanding of good nutrition boils down to learning about seven key subjects:

1. Protein
2. Dietary fat
3. Carbohydrate (including dietary fiber)
4. Water
5. Vitamins
6. Dietary minerals
7. Calories

Protein, dietary fat, carbohydrate, and water are called **macronutrients** ("large nutrients") because they are needed in large amounts. Vitamins and dietary minerals are termed **micronutrients** ("small nutrients") because they are needed in small amounts.

Protein

Protein is essential for growth, immune function, and the construction of hormones and enzymes. It is used to repair, maintain, and build the muscle fibers that are damaged during workouts, and can also act as an energy source in the absence of carbohydrate. To build muscle, you have to consume more protein than your body breaks down. An insufficient intake will result in slow strength and muscle gains or even loss of muscle.

Dietary fat

Dietary fat provides the most concentrated source of energy. It is vital for absorbing certain vitamins (A, D, E, and K), maintaining cell membranes, and building muscle. Fat plays a vital role in the manufacture of testosterone, which is important for promoting muscular growth and increasing strength. Fat may also help to increase levels of insulin-like growth factor 1 (IGF-1), another key hormone that stimulates growth in muscle and strength.

Carbohydrate

Carbohydrate is your body's main source of fuel. If you don't eat enough carbohydrate, when you exercise, you'll fatigue sooner, and your muscle and strength gains will be reduced. On the other hand, if you eat too much carbohydrate, it will be stored as fat.

Dietary fiber is a carbohydrate that is incompletely absorbed by your body. It helps to keep your digestive system healthy by increasing the size and weight of your stool and helping it to move through your digestive tract.

Water

Water makes up nearly two-thirds of your body. It is important for maintaining the balance of bodily fluids, which is essential for *every* function and chemical reaction that occurs within your body. For example, water is used to transport nutrients into, and waste products out of, cells. It is necessary for proper digestion, absorption, circulation, and excretion, as well as the assimilation of water-soluble vitamins. Water also helps to maintain proper body temperature. Because it is lost as sweat during exercise, water must be adequately replenished.

Vitamins

Vitamins are organic chemical compounds that the body can't synthesize in sufficient quantities and must therefore obtain from the diet. Common vitamins include vitamin D (which helps the body to absorb calcium, iron, magnesium, phosphate, and zinc from food) and vitamin C (which is important for proper growth and development, the maintenance of the immune system, and good vision).

Dietary minerals

Dietary minerals are inorganic chemical elements required by the body other than the four elements carbon, hydrogen, nitrogen, and oxygen. Some dietary minerals, such as iodine and fluoride, are only needed in tiny quantities. These are known as **trace elements**. Iodine is necessary for normal thyroid function and for the production of thyroid hormones. Fluoride helps to prevent tooth decay.

Other dietary minerals, such as iron and calcium, are needed in larger amounts. These are known as **macrominerals**. Iron is essential for numerous processes, including making the oxygen-carrying proteins **hemoglobin** and **myoglobin**. Calcium is important for strong bones and teeth.

Calories

Calories are the units of energy found in nutrients. Your body needs a certain number of calories each day to fuel bodily functions and physical activities. If you consume fewer calories than your body needs, you will lose weight; if you consume more calories than your body needs, you will gain weight. Therefore, being aware of the number of calories you take in is important and can help you to manage your weight.

Let's now look at everything just summarized in much more detail (except water and calories. Calories and calorie requirements will be explored in detail in the next chapter).

Protein

Why is protein important for weight training?

Protein is essential for repairing and building muscle, as well as maintaining muscle when dieting. **Amino acids**, which are the building blocks of proteins, are used to repair and build muscle fibers after they have been damaged by workouts. More specifically, the amino acids are used to repair and build new **actin** and **myosin** contractile protein filaments.

When you train, you stimulate an increase in the uptake of amino acids from your bloodstream. If amino acid quantities are insufficient, or if certain types of amino acid are missing, your body's ability to repair and build muscle tissue will be impaired. As a result, you will experience slow strength and muscle gains, or even muscle loss.

Protein is also used as an energy source. However, it is used as **anaerobic fuel** only when carbohydrates are low, or as **aerobic fuel** only when both carbohydrate and lipid (fat) resources are low.

What are the best sources of protein?

Protein can come from both animal and plant sources. Animal sources of protein include meats (chicken, beef, pork, turkey, fish, seafood, etc.), dairy products, and eggs. Plant sources include grains, nuts, legumes, peas, broccoli, and spinach.

However, not all sources of protein are the same. Some foods provide a better source of protein. The quality of a protein depends on its **amino acid content**.

Amino acids are the building blocks of proteins. There are **20** types of amino acid. Nine of them (leucine, lysine, threonine, isoleucine, phenylalanine, valine, methionine, tryptophan, and histidine) are termed **essential amino acids** (**EAAs**) because the body can't make them. EAAs must be obtained from your diet. The remaining 11 amino acids (arginine, cysteine, glycine, glutamine, proline, tyrosine, alanine, aspartic acid, asparagine, glutamic acid, and serine) can usually be made by your body using other amino acids. They are called **non-essential amino acids**.

When a protein contains EAAs in a proportion similar to that required by the body, it is said to have a high **biological value** (**BV**). When one or more of the EAAs are missing or present in low numbers, the protein is said to have a low BV. This means that the BV of a food is determined not only by the amino acid composition but also by the amount of the limiting amino acid (the amino acid present in the smallest quantity).

Keeping this in mind, the general advice is to consume:

- proteins that have a high BV
- a mixture of proteins.

Consuming a mixture of protein-rich foods and not just protein-rich foods that have a high BV is important because the limiting amino acid tends to be different in different foods. The shortfall in one type of amino acid in one food can be compensated by higher amounts of the amino acid in another food, thus producing a combination with a higher BV.

The importance of leucine

While all EAAs are important, **leucine** is a particularly important EAA for weight training. It is one of three amino acids known as **branched-chain amino acids** (**BCAAs**), and is unique in its ability to stimulate muscle protein synthesis. In fact, leucine may have up to ten times more of an impact on muscle protein synthesis than any other amino acid, making it very important for the recovery and growth of muscles after exercise. Rich sources of leucine include milk and whey.

How much protein do you need per day?

There is no one-size-fits-all answer to this question. Everybody is unique. However, there are some general guidelines with which you can start, after which you can make adjustments based on your results.

The amount of protein you need per day mainly depends on whether you are **bulking, cutting,** or **maintaining,** which are explained in detail in **Bulking and cutting,** in the next chapter. Most gym-goers will tell you that you need 1.0 gram of protein per pound of body weight per day (2.2 grams per kilogram of body weight per day) when bulking or maintaining, or you need up to 1.5 grams of protein per pound of body weight per day when cutting. These are longstanding recommendations, going back decades and used by many renowned bodybuilders. However, the current scientific consensus is that you only need **0.59 to 0.82** grams per pound of body weight per day (1.3 to 1.8 grams per kilogram of body weight per day) when bulking or maintaining, or **0.82 to 0.91** grams per pound of body weight per day (1.8 to 2.0

grams per kilogram of body weight per day) when cutting. If you're obese (have a body-mass index of 30 or more), then swap grams per **body weight** for grams per **fat-free body mass**, since the number of grams of protein that you will have to eat if calculated based on total body weight will be excessive.

Note, however, that you do not have to concern yourself too much with any of these figures. The reason is that, as explained in **Bulking and cutting**, you will be tracking your diet using an app. Once you input the recommended settings, the app will guide you to eating the right amount of protein.

What factors affect how much protein you need?

The amount of protein you need isn't just affected by whether you are bulking, cutting, or maintaining. Other factors can have small effects, which you should take into consideration if you ever have/want to make adjustments to your app settings:

- Fat-free body mass — the more fat-free or lean body mass you have, the more protein you will need.
- Training intensity — the harder you train, the higher your protein turnover will be, and therefore the more protein you will need.
- Weight training experience — the more years you have spent weight training, the less protein you will need because the better your body will have become at conserving protein (breaking down fewer proteins during exercise).
- Gender — Since the rate of protein synthesis is lower in women than it is in men, women need less protein than men do.

How much protein to eat per meal

It's recommended that you divide your daily protein requirement between your meals and do not concentrate all of your protein into one or two meals.

Eating protein before and after exercise

Consuming protein both before and after a workout could improve muscle protein synthesis. See **Nutrient timing** in the next chapter to learn more.

Protein supplements

Protein supplements are essential to help you get enough protein without consuming too much fat. See **Weight training supplements** in the next chapter for a discussion on protein and other supplements.

Dietary fat

Why is dietary fat important for weight training?

Fat is an essential part of your diet. It provides an important source of fuel, helps your body to absorb fat-soluble vitamins (A, D, E, and K), cushions your organs, insulates your body, and is used to build the cell membrane of every cell in your body. In the context of weight training, fat plays a vital role in the manufacture of testosterone, which is important for promoting muscle growth. Fat may also help to increase levels of insulin-like growth factor 1 (IGF-1), another key hormone that stimulates growth in muscle mass and strength.

Different types of dietary fat

There are two main types of dietary fat:

1. Unsaturated
2. Saturated

All foods that contain fat will provide a mixture of both unsaturated and saturated fats. However, unsaturated fats occur in higher amounts in plant products, whereas saturated fats occur in higher quantities in animal products.

Unsaturated fats

Unsaturated fats are liquid at room temperature. They can be broken down into three groups:

1. Monounsaturated fats
2. Polyunsaturated fats
3. Trans fats

Monounsaturated fats

Monounsaturated fats are considered healthy when eaten in moderation. They can lower your risk of heart disease and stroke by reducing the level of "bad" cholesterol in your blood. They also help to develop and maintain your body's cells. Monounsaturated fats can be found in avocados, peanut oil, olive oil, canola oil, almonds, peanuts, hazelnuts, pecans, cashews, pumpkin seeds, and sesame seeds.

Polyunsaturated fats

Like monounsaturated fats, polyunsaturated fats are considered healthy when consumed in moderation. They, too, help to lower the level of "bad" cholesterol in your blood, and are required to develop and maintain your body's cells. Polyunsaturated fats can be found in fish, fish oil, safflower oil, soybean oil, corn oil, canola oil, flaxseed oil, flaxseeds, and walnuts.

Two types of polyunsaturated fat, known as **alpha-linoleic acid** and **linoleic acid**, are very important because they cannot be made by the body and must therefore come from the diet. Alpha-linoleic acid is an **omega-3 fatty acid** and is used to make other omega-3 fatty acids; linoleic acid is an **omega-6 fatty acid** and is used to make other omega-6 fatty acids.

Omega-3 fatty acids are important for proper function of your nervous system, including your brain. Omega-3s also help to regulate hormones, ease inflammation, and reduce the risk of cardiovascular disease and stroke. In the context of weight training and exercise, omega-3 fatty acids increase the delivery of oxygen to muscles, improve aerobic capacity and endurance, speed up recovery, and reduce joint stiffness. Foods high in alpha-linoleic acid include fish (salmon, mackerel, and tuna), vegetable oils, nuts (especially walnuts), flaxseeds, flaxseed oil, and leafy vegetables.

As with omega-3 fatty acids, omega-6 fatty acids play a crucial role in the function of your nervous system. They also help to stimulate the growth of skin and hair, maintain the health of your bones, regulate your metabolism, and maintain your reproductive system. Foods high in omega-6 fatty acids include nuts, seeds, and plant oils, such as corn oil, soybean oil, and sunflower oil.

A healthy diet should contain a balance of omega-3 and omega-6 fatty acids in a **1:1 ratio**. One of the reasons is that omega-3 fatty acids help to reduce inflammation, whereas some omega-6 fatty acids tend to promote inflammation. The problem is that omega-6 fatty acids are more widely found in modern foods than omega-3 fatty acids. The typical American tends to consume 14 to 25 times more omega-6 than omega-3! Consuming an excessive amount of omega-6 relative to omega-3 for a prolonged period, as many people do in the developed world, is believed by some to be a contributory factor to the prevalence of chronic inflammation, cancer, neurodegenerative disease, heart attack, stroke, and many of the other common health problems in the developed world.

Trans fats

Trans fats are considered very unhealthy and should be avoided. They are known to raise bad cholesterol levels and decrease good cholesterol levels (a combination that increases your risk of heart disease and stroke) even more than do saturated fats. Trans fats have also been associated with insulin resistance and inflammation.

Trans fats can be naturally occurring or artificial. Naturally occurring trans fats are produced in the gut of some animals, and can therefore be found in certain meats and dairy products. However, the quantity is small. Most of the trans fats in your diet come from artificial sources.

Artificial trans fats are made by adding hydrogen to liquid vegetable oils in an industrial process called **hydrogenation**, which makes the oil more solid and stable. This **partially hydrogenated oil**, as it is known, is less likely to spoil, so foods made with it have a longer shelf life. Partially hydrogenated oil is also used by some restaurants for deep frying because the oil can withstand repeated heating without breaking down and therefore doesn't have to be changed as often as other types of oil.

As a result of these "benefits", partially hydrogenated oils became popular in restaurants and the food industry, being used for frying and in the making of baked goods, processed snacks, and margarine. You are therefore most likely to find trans fats in processed or deep-fried foods, such as margarine, imitation cheese, cakes, cookies, doughnuts, crackers, and chips. Fortunately, trans fats are gradually being eliminated from many of these foods.

Food labels in the US are allowed to state that a food contains no trans fat if the amount is less than 0.5 grams. If you consume several servings of these foods, the hidden trans fat content can quickly add up. Therefore, in addition to the food label, you should check the ingredients for "partially hydrogenated vegetable oil", which will indicate whether the food contains some trans fat even if the amount is less than 0.5 grams.

Saturated fat

Saturated fats are solid at room temperature. They are mainly found in animal foods, such as red meat, whole milk, cheese, ice cream, yogurt, chocolate, butter, lard, seafood, and eggs (in the yolk). They also occur in some plant-based foods, such as coconut, coconut oil, palm oil, and palm kernel oil.

In the past, saturated fats were considered unhealthy because they were linked to an increase in bad cholesterol, which increases the risk of heart disease and stroke. However, that idea has started to change since certain studies have found a lack of evidence. Even so, the message remains that cutting back on saturated fats can be good for health, especially if replaced with monounsaturated fats.

How much fat do you need per day?

The *2015–2020 Dietary Guidelines for Americans*, published by the US Department of Health and Human Services and the US Department of Agriculture (USDA), recommends that 20% to 35% of the daily kilocalories consumed by men and women aged 19 and over should come from fat. Just make sure that you favor foods that are high in unsaturated fat, limit foods that are high in saturated fat, and completely avoid foods that contain trans fat (which may be listed in the food's ingredients as "partially hydrogenated vegetable oil"). Also, try to get an equal and sufficient amount of omega-3 and omega-6.

Carbohydrate and dietary fiber

Why is carbohydrate important for weight training?

Carbohydrate is your body's main source of fuel. Generally speaking, when you eat carbohydrate, the digestible parts are broken down into the sugar **glucose**, which provides energy for the cells of your body. Any remaining glucose is stored in a form known as **glycogen** in your liver and in muscle cells for later use. If glycogen stores are full, excess glucose is stored as fat. All of this means that if you don't consume enough carbohydrate, your workouts (and therefore your gains) will be compromised. You'll fatigue sooner when you train, and your muscle and strength gains will be reduced. Conversely, if you regularly eat too much carbohydrate, the excess will be added to your waistline (men) or hips, butt, and thighs (women).

Since carbohydrate stimulates the release of insulin, it's also important for building muscle. Insulin allows amino acids and glucose to enter muscle cells, where they can be used for energy, muscular repair, and muscular growth. Without insulin, your muscle cells will not be able to use amino acids or glucose.

Another way in which carbohydrate affects muscular development is through its effect on **testosterone** and **cortisol** (a stress hormone that is associated with muscle breakdown). Low-carbohydrate diets are known to decrease the level of testosterone and increase the level of cortisol.

Types of carbohydrate

There are four types of carbohydrate, which are classified based on their molecular complexity:

1. Monosaccharides
2. Disaccharides
3. Oligosaccharides
4. Polysaccharides

Monosaccharides and disaccharides are known as **simple carbohydrates** or **sugars**, whereas oligosaccharides and polysaccharides are known as **complex carbohydrates**.

Monosaccharides ("single sugars") are the most basic units of carbohydrate. They cannot be broken down any further, and include glucose (also known as dextrose), fructose (fruit sugar), and galactose (found in dairy products). Monosaccharides are the building blocks of disaccharides, oligosaccharides, and polysaccharides.

Disaccharides ("double sugars") are formed of two monosaccharides. They include sucrose (table sugar), maltose (malt sugar), and lactose (milk sugar).

Oligosaccharides ("a few sugars") are composed of three to ten monosaccharides. The more complex oligosaccharides cannot be digested by the body, and therefore act as **fiber**. Fiber, as described in more detail below, is any plant-based food material that cannot be fully digested.

Oligosaccharides offer a variety of health benefits, including helping to feed friendly bacteria (known as **probiotics**) in the large intestine. These kinds of oligosaccharides are known as **prebiotics**. Two common oligosaccharides are raffinose and stachyose, which are found in beans and other legumes. As probiotics break them down, the gas for which beans are famous is produced.

Polysaccharides ("many sugars") are chains containing more than ten monosaccharide units. Examples include starch, glycogen, cellulose, and chitin. Starch, which is composed simply of glucose, is the only digestible polysaccharide. It can be found in grains, root vegetables, and legumes.

Dietary fiber

Dietary fiber can be found only in plant products, such as nuts, whole grains, legumes, fruits, and vegetables. It can be defined as any plant-based food material that cannot be fully digested. However, despite being mostly indigestible, dietary fiber is still extremely important for your health, helping to reduce the risk of heart disease, cancer, infectious diseases, and respiratory illnesses, as well as promote healthy bowel movements (**laxation**). Fiber also aids weight loss by reducing food intake. This is because fiber-rich foods take longer to digest and therefore lead to an increased feeling of fullness and satiety.

There are two types of dietary fiber:

1. Soluble
2. Insoluble

Soluble fiber dissolves in water, swells, and forms a gel-like substance, some of which is digested and absorbed. The gradual absorption slows the entrance of glucose into the blood stream, thereby preventing large blood glucose and insulin spikes. Soluble fibers include pectins, gums, mucilages, and some hemicelluloses. Good sources of soluble fiber include oats, peas, beans, lentils, barley, fruits, and vegetables, especially carrots, apples, and oranges.

Insoluble fiber does not dissolve in water. It passes through your digestive tract in close to its original structure, which adds weight and size to your stool and therefore aids bowel movements. This offers many benefits to intestinal health, including a reduction in the risk of hemorrhoids and constipation. Insoluble fibers include cellulose, lignins, and some hemicelluloses.

Most insoluble fibers come from the bran layers of cereal grains. Whole-wheat flour, whole grains, wheat bran, and brown rice are full of insoluble fiber. It can also be found in the seeds and skins of fruits, so always eat your peels!

As published in the *2015–2020 Dietary Guidelines for Americans*, the USDA recommends a fiber intake of 28 grams per day for women aged 19 and over, or 34 grams per day for men aged 19 and over. This should include a combination of both soluble and insoluble fiber. The average American consumes on average only 15 grams of fiber per day, which falls far short of the recommended amount. You can increase the amount of fiber that you ingest by making simple changes to your dietary habits, such as:

- choosing whole fruits and vegetables instead of juices
- consuming fruits and vegetables without peeling them (if possible)
- choosing whole-grain breads, cereals, and pastas over processed and refined varieties
- choosing goods made with whole-wheat flour instead of white flour
- swapping white rice for brown rice
- occasionally replacing meat with beans or other legumes.

What are the best sources of carbohydrate?

The best sources of carbohydrate are nutrient-dense and fiber-rich whole foods, such as whole-wheat breads and pastas, brown rice, porridge, sweet potato, legumes, fruits, and vegetables. Many individuals think it's important to only eat carbohydrates that have a low **glycemic index**; however, that is unwise.

The Glycemic Index

The Glycemic Index (GI) is a measure of how rapidly a food containing 50 grams of carbohydrate will make your blood glucose level rise after consumption. Pure glucose has the highest GI of 100. All foods containing carbohydrate are given a score between 0 and 100, and are ranked as either low, medium, or high based on their score. Two foods with the same amount of carbohydrate can have different GIs. The higher the food's GI is, the faster the carbohydrate content can be broken down and absorbed, causing a rapid increase in blood glucose.

Consistently high blood glucose levels or repeated blood glucose "spikes" following a meal may increase an individual's chances of developing type 2 diabetes and coronary heart disease, which is why high-GI foods are generally not recommended. However, it's important to note that the GI of a food is based on eating the food by itself. When eaten with other foods, the meal's overall GI will be different. Combining high-GI foods with low-GI foods will balance out the effect on blood glucose levels. Fat, fiber, and acidic foods (such as lemon juice or vinegar) help to lower the GI of a meal. Other factors that may affect a food's GI include:

- ripeness — the riper a fruit or vegetable is, the higher its GI may be
- processing — the more processed a food is, the higher its GI may be
- cooking method — the longer a food is cooked, the higher its GI may be.

Another important point to note is that many nutritious foods have a higher GI than foods that lack nutritional value. For example, wholemeal bread has a higher GI than a Mars bar! Therefore, judging a food solely based on its GI isn't wise and should be balanced with other principles of nutrition, such as moderating foods that have low nutritional value.

How much carbohydrate do you need per day?

The USDA recommends in the *2015–2020 Dietary Guidelines for Americans* that 45% to 65% of the daily kilocalories consumed by males and females of any age should come from carbohydrate. Since carbohydrate is your main source of fuel, the more active you are, the more carbohydrate you will need to fuel your activities. However, keep sugars to a minimum (less than 10% of your daily caloric intake).

Vitamins

What are vitamins?

Vitamins are organic chemical compounds that your body needs but cannot synthesize in sufficient quantities by itself. They have diverse biochemical functions and are very important for proper health, growth, metabolism, and function.

Together with dietary minerals, vitamins are known as **micronutrients** because they are needed by the body in small amounts. In comparison, **macronutrients** (protein, carbohydrate, and fat) are needed in large amounts.

You can get all of the vitamins you need from your diet, provided it is balanced, nutrient-dense, and varied. If you do not get enough of a certain vitamin, you may suffer from health problems. Vitamin deficiencies can be fixed by changing your diet or taking a supplement. Before starting a supplement, speak to your doctor. It is better to consume a variety of foods instead of taking a multivitamin supplement because the supplement may not be absorbed properly. You can also suffer from health problems if you get too much of a vitamin for a prolonged period of time.

Types of vitamin

There are 13 types of vitamin:

- Vitamin A
- Vitamin C
- Vitamin D
- Vitamin E
- Vitamin K
- B vitamins (thiamine, riboflavin, niacin, pantothenic acid, vitamin B6, biotin, folate, and vitamin B12)

According to the USDA, adult Americans do not typically get enough of vitamins A, C, and E. Vegetarians may also need to supplement vitamin B12.

Vitamin A

Vitamin A is needed for good vision, and the proper growth and maintenance of your cells. Good sources of vitamin A include:

- Vegetables, such as sweet potato, sweet red pepper, carrots, and lettuce
- Dark leafy greens, such as kale, spinach, dandelion greens, collards, Swiss chard, and pak choi
- Fruits, such as butternut squash, pumpkin, cantaloupe, mango, and papaya
- Dried apricots, dried prunes, and dried peaches
- Fishes, such as tuna, sturgeon, and mackerel

- Oysters

Vitamin C

Vitamin C helps the body to form **collagen**, which is the main protein used as connective tissue in the body. Good sources of vitamin C include:

- Fruits, such as guava, oranges, kiwis, strawberries, cantaloupe, papaya, pineapple, and mango
- Vegetables, such as raw red sweet pepper, raw green sweet pepper, Brussels sprouts, broccoli, sweet potatoes, and cauliflower

Vitamin D

Vitamin D is responsible for enhancing your body's absorption of the minerals calcium, iron, magnesium, phosphate, and zinc. It is synthesized in small amounts by your body when ultraviolet rays from sunlight strike your skin, but you should also get some through your diet. Vitamin D is naturally present in very few foods. Consequently, it is often artificially added to foods, such as milk, breakfast cereals, juices, yogurts, and margarines. Natural sources of vitamin D include:

- Fatty fishes, such as salmon, tuna, and mackerel
- Fish liver oils
- Beef liver
- Cheese
- Egg yolks
- Mushrooms

Vitamin E

Vitamin E is an **antioxidant**, which is a nutrient that helps fight damage to the cells in the body. Good sources of vitamin E include:

- Nuts and seeds, such as sunflower seeds, almonds, hazelnuts, pine nuts, peanuts, and brazil nuts
- Turnip greens
- Peanut butter
- Spinach
- Avocado
- Tomato paste, sauce, and puree

Vitamin K

Vitamin K plays a key role in helping your blood to clot, which prevents excessive bleeding. It's also needed for strong bones. Vitamin K is generally not supplemented. You should not take vitamin K supplements unless your doctor tells you to do so. Good natural sources of vitamin K include:

- Leafy green vegetables, such as spinach, cabbage, Swiss chard, lettuce, kale, cauliflower, broccoli, dandelion greens, and Brussels sprouts
- Some fruits, such as avocados, kiwis, strawberries, and grapes
- Some vegetable oils, such as soybean oil

B vitamins

There are eight B vitamins:

1. Thiamine (vitamin B1)
2. Riboflavin (vitamin B2)
3. Niacin (vitamin B3)
4. Pantothenic acid (vitamin B5)
5. Vitamin B6
6. Biotin (vitamin B7)
7. Folate (vitamin B9)
8. Vitamin B12

B vitamins are needed for healthy skin, hair, and eyes, as well as healthy liver and nervous system function. All of them also help your body to convert carbohydrates into glucose, as well as metabolize fats and proteins.

Thiamine (vitamin B1) is needed to form **adenosine triphosphate** (**ATP**), which every cell in your body uses for energy. Good dietary sources of thiamine include:

- Legumes, such as beans and lentils
- Meats, such as beef and pork
- Brewer's yeast
- Whole-grain breads and cereals
- Oatmeal
- Rice bran and wheat germ
- Milk

Riboflavin (vitamin B2) helps your body to utilize the other B vitamins. It may also help to protect cells from oxidative damage. Good sources of riboflavin include:

- Meats, such as lamb, beef liver, and wild salmon
- Milk and yogurt
- Eggs
- Mushrooms
- Spinach
- Almonds
- Sun-dried tomatoes

Niacin (vitamin B3) is essential for processing fat in the body, lowering cholesterol, and regulating blood sugar. Good sources of niacin include:

- Fishes, such as tuna, mackerel, and skipjack
- Other meats, such as pork, chicken, beef, turkey, and liver
- Peanuts
- Green peas
- Sunflower seeds
- Avocados

Pantothenic acid (vitamin B5) is essential for cellular processes and optimal maintenance of fat. Good sources of pantothenic acid include:

- Meats, such as pork, beef, chicken, turkey, and oily fish (e.g. trout and wild salmon)
- Eggs
- Cheese
- Mushrooms
- Avocados
- Sweet potatoes
- Sunflower seeds

Vitamin B6 is necessary for the proper maintenance of red blood cell metabolism, the nervous system, the immune system, and many other bodily functions. Good sources include:

- Fishes, such as wild salmon, halibut, and tuna
- Meats, such as turkey, chicken, and lean beef and pork
- Dried fruits, such as apricots, prunes, and raisins
- Sunflower seeds
- Pistachio nuts
- Bananas
- Avocados
- Cooked spinach

Biotin (vitamin B7) plays a central role in many pathways of metabolism, including fat and sugar metabolism. The best sources of biotin are:

- Meats, such as salmon, pork, and liver
- Yeast and whole-wheat bread
- Various nuts, such as almonds and walnuts
- Some types of berries, including strawberries and raspberries
- Vegetables, such as Swiss chard, carrots, onions, cucumbers, and cauliflower
- Egg yolk
- Milk

- Tofu
- Mushrooms

Folate (vitamin B9) is required for numerous bodily functions, including DNA synthesis and repair, cellular division, and cell growth. Folate is especially important in pregnant women, in whom it is used for proper fetal development. Folic acid is the synthetic form of **folate**, found in fortified foods and supplements. Good, natural sources of folate include:

- Beans, such as black-eyed peas, mung beans, pinto beans, and chickpeas
- Lentils
- Vegetables, such as spinach, asparagus, lettuce, and broccoli
- Tropical fruits, such as mango, pomegranate, papaya, guava, kiwi, and banana
- Avocados
- Oranges
- Wheat bread

Vitamin B12 is the largest and most complex vitamin. It can only be synthesized by bacteria and can only be found naturally in animal products. Synthetic vitamin B12 is widely available and added to many foods, such as cereals. Good natural sources include:

- Shellfish, such as oysters and mussels
- Beef and chicken liver
- Fishes, such as tuna, mackerel, salmon, herring, and sardines
- Crab, shrimp, and crayfish
- Meats, such as beef and lamb
- Low-fat milk and yogurt
- Swiss cheese
- Eggs

Dietary minerals

What are dietary minerals?

Dietary minerals are inorganic chemical elements that your body needs for proper health, growth, and function. Along with vitamins, dietary minerals are known as **micronutrients** because they are needed by the body in small amounts. **Macronutrients**, in comparison (which include protein, carbohydrate, and fat), are needed in large amounts.

Your body uses minerals for many different jobs, including building bones and making hormones. You can get all of the dietary minerals you need from your diet, as long as it is balanced, nutrient-dense, and diverse. If you do not consume enough of a certain mineral, you may suffer from health problems. Mineral deficiencies can be fixed by modifying your diet or taking a supplement. Before taking a supplement, speak to your doctor. You can also suffer from health problems if you get too much of a mineral.

Types of dietary minerals

Dietary minerals are classified into two groups based on how much your body needs:

1. Macrominerals
2. Trace minerals

Macrominerals are minerals your body needs in relatively large amounts. They include:

- Calcium
- Potassium
- Magnesium
- Phosphorus
- Sodium
- Chloride
- Sulfur

Trace minerals are minerals your body needs in relatively small amounts. They include:

- Iron
- Manganese
- Copper
- Iodine
- Zinc
- Selenium
- Chromium
- Fluoride

According to the USDA, adult Americans typically do not get enough calcium, potassium, and magnesium, with potassium being deficient the most.

Macrominerals

<u>Calcium</u>

Calcium is the most abundant mineral in your body. Your body needs calcium to build strong bones and teeth, and to maintain strong and healthy bones. The following foods are good sources of calcium:

- Low-fat yogurt, cheese, and milk
- Fishes, such as sardines, pink salmon, and ocean perch
- Beans, such as soybeans and white beans

- Spinach
- Oatmeal

Potassium

Potassium is a very important dietary mineral, used by your body to build proteins (and therefore muscle), maintain normal body growth, break down carbohydrates, control the electrical activity of your heart, and maintain a healthy blood pressure. Good sources of potassium include:

- Fishes, such as halibut, yellowfin tuna, rockfish, and cod
- Beans, such as white beans, soybeans, lima beans, and kidney beans
- Milk and dairy products, such as yogurt
- Sweet and regular potatoes
- Fruits, such as bananas, peaches, cantaloupe, and honeydew melons
- Tomato paste, puree, juice, and sauce

Magnesium

Magnesium helps your body to produce energy, and helps your muscles, arteries, and heart to work properly. Good sources of magnesium are:

- Vegetables, such as pumpkin, spinach, and artichoke
- Bran cereal
- Beans, such as soybeans, white beans, black beans, navy beans, and great northern beans
- Tofu
- Brown rice
- Nuts, such as brazil nuts, almonds, cashews, and peanuts

Phosphorus

After calcium, phosphorus is the second most abundant mineral in your body. Your body needs phosphorus for a variety of purposes, such as building strong bones and teeth, filtering waste from your kidneys, managing the usage and storage of energy, repairing tissues, ensuring proper nerve signalling, and utilizing certain vitamins and minerals (vitamin B, vitamin D, iodine, magnesium, and zinc). In the context of weight training and exercise, phosphorus is important for assisting muscle contraction and reducing muscle soreness after exercise.

Most foods contain phosphorus. As a result, you're more likely to get too much than too little. Foods that are rich in protein are also usually rich in phosphorus. These include:

- Meats and poultry
- Fishes
- Milk and dairy products
- Eggs
- Nuts and seeds

- Beans

Sodium

Sodium is important for controlling the balance of fluid in your body, and maintaining your blood volume and blood pressure. The problem is that you may already be getting too much, which could lead to high blood pressure and fluid retention.

The main source of sodium for most people is table salt (**sodium chloride**). The average American takes in five or more teaspoons of table salt per day, when, in fact, only one quarter of a teaspoon is needed. Sodium also naturally occurs in foods, and a lot of it is often artificially added to foods during processing and preparation. Large amounts can be found in canned and fast foods.

Chloride

Chloride is needed to control the balance of bodily fluids and is an essential part of digestive juices. As with sodium, it is consumed, often in excess, mainly though table salt. Getting too much chloride from salted foods can lead to high blood pressure and fluid retention. Chloride also occurs naturally in many vegetables. Foods with high amounts of chloride include:

- Seaweed
- Rye
- Tomatoes
- Lettuce
- Celery
- Olives

Sulphur

Sulphur helps your body to resist bacteria and protect against toxic substances. It is also necessary for proper development of connective tissues and helps skin maintain structural integrity. Good sources of sulphur include:

- Cruciferous vegetables, such as cauliflower, Brussels sprouts, broccoli, kale, cabbage, and turnips
- Allium vegetables, such as garlic, onions, leeks, and chives
- Meats, such as beef, fish, and poultry
- Nuts
- Legumes
- Egg whites

Trace minerals

Iron

Iron is important for the production of proteins called **hemoglobin** and **myoglobin**. The former is found in red blood cells, whereas the latter is found in muscle cells. Hemoglobin and myoglobin are very important because they bind to oxygen, carry it around your body, and deliver it to cells. Iron also supports immune function, temperature regulation, and brain development.

There are two types of dietary iron: **heme** and **non-heme**. Heme iron is derived from hemoglobin, which means that it comes from animal sources that originally contained hemoglobin. Non-heme iron comes from plant sources. Heme iron is absorbed by your body more readily than is non-heme iron. Great sources of heme iron include:

- Meats, such as beef, turkey, chicken, ham, beef liver, and chicken liver
- Shellfish, such as clams, mussels, and oysters
- Fishes, such as sardines, halibut, haddock, perch, salmon, and tuna

Manganese

Manganese is required for the production of bones, connective tissues, skin, and sex hormones. It's also used for the regulation of blood sugar, the absorption of calcium, and the breakdown of dietary fats and carbohydrates. Foods high in manganese include:

- Seafood, such as mussels, clams, and crayfish
- Nuts, such as hazelnuts, walnuts, macadamia, cashew nuts, and almonds
- Seeds, such as sesame seeds, flaxseeds, and sunflower seeds
- Whole-wheat bread
- Tofu
- Beans, such as butter beans, winged beans, chickpeas, adzuki beans, and white beans
- Fishes, such as bass, pike, and perch
- Spinach
- Brown rice

Copper

Copper is needed by your body to produce bones, connective tissues, enzymes, and important neurotransmitters. In order to absorb copper, your stomach has to be acidic. As such, **antacids** can interfere with the absorption of copper, as can milk and egg proteins. Good sources of copper include:

- Seafood, such as oysters, lobsters, crabs, and octopuses
- Raw kale
- Mushrooms
- Various seeds, such as sesame seeds, pumpkin seeds, squash seeds, and flaxseeds
- Nuts, such as hazelnuts, brazil nuts, cashew nuts, walnuts, pine nuts, and pistachio nuts
- Beans, such as soybeans, adzuki beans, kidney beans, and white beans
- Dried fruits, such as apricots, currents, peaches, raisins, and figs
- Avocados

Iodine

The only cells in your body that absorb iodine are in you thyroid. Your thyroid uses iodine to produce two hormones: **triiodothyronine** (T3) and **thyroxine** (T4). T3 and T4 are primarily responsible for the regulation of your metabolism, which makes them extremely important. A lack of iodine in your diet can lead to a decreased production of T3 and T4. Although vital, your body only needs 150 micrograms (one-20,000[th] of a teaspoon) of iodine per day. Common sources of iodine include:

- Dairy products, such as cheese, cow's milk, yogurt, ice cream
- Seaweed, including kelp, dulce, and nori
- Saltwater fish
- Shellfish
- Eggs
- Iodized table salt
- Soy milk and soy sauce

Zinc

Zinc is found throughout your body. It is required for maintaining a proper sense of taste and smell, and helps your immune system to fight invading bacteria and viruses. Your body also needs zinc to make proteins and DNA, and heal wounds.

Zinc is found in a variety of foods. Rich sources include:

- Oysters, which are the best source of zinc
- Other seafood, such as crabs and lobsters
- Meats, such as beef, lamb, pork, chicken, and poultry
- Wheat germ
- Spinach
- Seeds, such as pumpkin seeds and squash seeds
- Nuts, such as cashew nuts, pecan nuts, pine nuts, almonds, walnuts, and peanuts
- Cocoa and chocolate (yippee!)
- Beans, such as chickpeas, baked beans, adzuki beans, and kidney beans

Selenium

Selenium is required by the body for proper thyroid gland function. It is also used to produce **selenoprotein antioxidants**, which are compounds that protect your cells from damage caused by negatively charged particles. High-selenium foods include:

- Nuts, such as brazil nuts, cashew nuts, black walnuts, and macadamia nuts
- Seafood, such as oysters, mussels, octopuses, squids, lobsters, and clams
- Fishes, such as tuna, rockfish, swordfish, halibut, tilapia, mackerel, and snapper
- Whole-wheat bread
- Seeds, such as sunflower seeds, chia seeds, sesame seeds, flaxseeds, and pumpkin seeds

- Meats, such as pork, beef, lamb, chicken, and turkey
- Mushrooms
- Whole grains, such as brown rice and rye

Chromium

Chromium is an important dietary mineral for your body's metabolism. It enhances the action of insulin, the hormone that regulates the breakdown and storage of carbohydrates, fats, and proteins in your body. Good sources of chromium include:

- Meats, such as beef and turkey
- Vegetables, such as broccoli, potatoes, and basil
- Fruits, such as apples, grapes, and bananas
- Red wine
- Green beans
- Garlic
- Whole-wheat bread

Fluoride

Fluoride can be found naturally in your body as **calcium fluoride**, which mostly occurs in your bones and teeth. You only need a small amount of fluoride each day to keep your bones strong and to prevent tooth decay.

Fluoride can be obtained in two ways: **topically** and **systemically**. Topical fluoride sources include toothpastes and mouthwashes, which are used to strengthen teeth that are already formed in your mouth. Systemic fluorides are those that are ingested, usually through drinking water, and become incorporated into developing teeth and bones.

The fluoride content of foods is very low. Fluoride has been added to the US water supply since the 1960s. If you brush your teeth with fluoride toothpaste and live in an area where the water has been **fluoridated**, you most likely get more than enough fluoride in your diet.

Chapter 6: Dietary management and strategic eating

Calories and calorie requirements

Now that we've gone over all of the macronutrients and micronutrients and have a basic foundation in nutrition, we can start to explore how nutrition can be managed and used to meet our weight training and fitness objectives. Arguably the most powerful and useful tool when it comes to managing and manipulating your diet is the process of counting calories.

What are calories?

Calories are the units of energy found in foods. Your body needs calories to fuel bodily functions and your physical activity. You get most of your calories from the **macronutrients** (carbohydrate, protein, and fat) that you eat. The calories are expressed in **kilocalories** (kcal). When people talk about calories, they usually mean kilocalories. One gram of carbohydrate provides four kilocalories, as does one gram of protein, whereas one gram of fat provides nine kilocalories.

What is basal metabolic rate?

Your basal metabolic rate (BMR) is the number of kilocalories your body needs each day at rest. In other words, it's the number of kilocalories your body needs just to maintain normal bodily functions, such as circulation, respiration, and temperature regulation. It does not include any physical activity.

BMR is very difficult to physically measure accurately. It requires a trip to a sophisticated lab, and lots of preparation, including approximately 12 hours of fasting to ensure that your digestive system is no longer active.

What is resting daily energy expenditure?

Resting daily energy expenditure (RDEE) is a less strict and less accurate measure of the number of kilocalories your body burns at rest. It is often used instead of BMR in scientific experiments because it is easier to physically measure (no need for fasting) and produces a value that is pretty close to your BMR. Because RDEE and BMR are so similar, they are often used interchangeably to mean the number of kilocalories your body burns at rest.

What is total daily energy expenditure?

Your total daily energy expenditure (TDEE) is the total number of kilocalories your body needs each day to fuel all of your bodily functions and all of your physical activity. Your TDEE is also known as your **maintenance calories**.

Why is your TDEE important when weight training?

The number of kilocalories you eat determines how your levels of fat and muscle might change as you train. Generally speaking:

- if you consistently consume fewer kilocalories than your TDEE, you will lose fat and maybe a little muscle
- if you consistently meet your TDEE, you will maintain your current level of fat (or maybe lose a little) and add muscle gradually
- if you consistently consume more kilocalories than your TDEE, you will optimize muscular growth but also gain fat.

Therefore, you can manipulate your caloric intake to promote these different goals.

For people who are completely new to weight training, the story is a little different. "Newbies" seem to be able to simultaneously gain muscle and lose fat almost no matter what they eat! However, as they become more experienced, gaining muscle and losing fat at the same time becomes increasingly difficult. At that point, as described above, they have to resort to phases of caloric surplus to optimize muscular growth (known as **bulking**) and phases of caloric deficit to lose fat (known as **cutting**). Bulking and cutting are explained in detail below.

How do you calculate your TDEE?

Thanks to the advent of apps, you no longer need to calculate your TDEE. All you have to do is use an app to track your diet, and the app will tell you if you are in a state of caloric deficit, maintenance, or surplus. I explain how to track your calories and diet later in this chapter, in **How to track your calories and diet**. However, just in case you want to know how to calculate your TDEE manually, I explain it below. If you don't want to know how to do it manually, you can move on to **Bulking and cutting**.

How to manually calculate your TDEE

There are a number of manual ways to calculate your TDEE. The most accurate formulas take your fat-free mass (also known as your **lean body mass**) into account. The most popular equation for calculating TDEE without knowing your lean body mass is the **Harris–Benedict formula**, and the most popular equation for calculating your TDEE using your lean body mass is the **Katch–McArdle formula**.

The Harris–Benedict formula

The Harris-Benedict formula of calculating TDEE involves two steps, one to calculate your BMR and another to multiply your BMR by an activity factor.

<u>Step 1</u>

Estimate your BMR. The formula is different for men and women.

Men: BMR = (10 x weight in kg) + (6.25 x height in cm) – (5 x age in years) + 5

Women: BMR = (10 x weight in kg) + (6.25 x height in cm) – (5 x age in years) – 161

Note: To convert pounds to kilograms, just divide the pounds by 2.2.

Step 2

Multiply your BMR by the appropriate activity factor in Table 6.1.

Level of physical activity	Activity factor
Sedentary (little or no exercise)	1.200
Lightly active (light exercise/sports 1–3 days/week)	1.375
Moderately active (moderate exercise/sports 3–5 days/week)	1.550
Very active (hard exercise/sports 6–7 days/week)	1.725
Extra active (hard daily exercise/sports and a physical job, or training twice daily)	1.900

Table 6.1. Levels of physical activity and their corresponding activity factors.

The resultant figure is your TDEE — that is, the number of kilocalories your body needs each day to maintain your current weight.

Note that by not taking lean body mass into account, the Harris–Benedict equation assumes that you have an average amount of lean body mass. As a result, it is accurate for most people but not for those who are very muscular or overweight. For very muscular individuals, it will underestimate caloric requirements because leaner bodies require more calories. For overweight individuals, it will overestimate caloric requirements because it will assume that the individual has more lean muscle mass than he or she actually has. Therefore, if you have more than average muscle mass, you can compensate by adding 150 kilocalories to your TDEE. Or, if you are obese, you can compensate by subtracting 150 kilocalories from your TDEE.

The Katch–McArdle formula

Unlike the Harris–Benedict formula, the Katch–McArdle formula does require that you know your lean body mass. Because it takes lean body mass into account, it can be more accurate than the Harris–Benedict formula, especially for people who are very muscular or overweight.

The Katch–McArdle formula of calculating TDEE is the same for both men and women and involves two steps, one to calculate your RDEE and another to multiply your RDEE by an activity factor. Remember that your RDEE is practically the same as your BMR.

Note: I explained how to work out your body-fat percentage in the **Weight Training Guide**, in **How to track your progress**.

Step 1

Calculate your RDEE. The formula looks like this:

RDEE = 370 + (21.6 x lean body mass in kilograms)

Or, if you want to work with pounds:

RDEE = 370 + (9.79759519 x lean body mass in pounds)

You can work out your lean body mass by subtracting the weight of your body fat from your total body weight using this equation:

Lean body mass = (1 – body fat percentage expressed as a decimal numeral) x total body weight

For example, if you weigh 160 pounds and have 18% body fat, your equation would look like this:

1 – 0.18 = 0.82

0.82 x 160 = 131.2 lb of lean body mass

You can now plug your lean body mass into the above formula to get your RDEE, thus:

RDEE = 370 + (9.79759519 x 131.2) = 1,655

Step 2

Multiply your RDEE by the appropriate activity factor in Table 6.1. The resultant figure is your TDEE — that is, the number of kilocalories you have to consume each day to maintain your current weight.

The problem with the Katch–McArdle formula is that it does not take age into consideration. As a result, it has been known to overestimate the caloric requirements of elderly individuals. Therefore, if you are over 50, and especially if you are over 65, you can compensate by subtracting 5% from your TDEE, or simply use the Harris–Benedict formula instead to calculate caloric requirements.

Bulking and cutting

What are bulking and cutting?

Bulking and cutting are **nutritional cycles**. As mentioned above, "bulking" means to consume more kilocalories each day than your body needs — that is, to put your body into a state of **caloric surplus**. This state optimizes muscular growth. Unfortunately, it also leads to gaining some body fat.

"Cutting" means to consume fewer kilocalories each day than your body needs — that is, to put your body into a state of **caloric deficit**. The aim of cutting is to lose body fat without losing much muscle.

The origin of bulking and cutting was in bodybuilding. Bulking helps bodybuilders to gain muscle before a competition, and cutting helps them to get rid of the unwanted body fat and be left with a well-defined physique or figure before the competition.

There is also "maintaining", which means to consume the same number of kilocalories each day that your body needs. The purpose of maintaining is to retain your current physique or figure.

Should you bulk, cut, or maintain?

Whether you should bulk, cut, or maintain depends on your goal, training experience, and body-fat percentage. The American Council on Exercise (ACE) has provided the following body-fat percentage ranges (Table 6.2).

	Women (%)	Men (%)
Essential fat	10–13	2–5
Athlete	14–20	6–13
Fitness	21–24	14–17
Acceptable	25–31	18–24
Obese	32+	25+

Table 6.2. ACE body-fat percentage ranges. Essential fat is the minimum amount of fat necessary for basic physical and physiological health.

Note: I explained how to work out your body-fat percentage in the **Weight Training Guide**, in **How to track your progress**.

Assuming that you have little or no proper training experience and your goal is to maximize growth in strength and muscle (or curves if you're a lady), I'd generally recommend the following bulking and cutting guidelines.

- If your initial body-fat percentage falls within the Athlete range (that is, 6% to 13% for men and 14% to 20% for women), you can start with a bulk. If at any point your body-fat percentage exceeds the Fitness range, you should cut.
- If your initial body-fat percentage falls within the Fitness or Acceptable ranges, you can start by maintaining. Together with a healthy diet and an effective training program, you should lose fat and build muscle/curves at the same time. Your goal will be to bring your body-fat percentage down to the Athlete range, after which you can bulk. If you fall short of achieving the range, get some assistance from a cut.
- If your initial body-fat percentage is in the Obese range, you should start with a cut. Your goal will be to bring your body-fat percentage down to the Athlete range, after which you can bulk. By then, you should have already built a significant amount of muscle/curves.
- When you're happy with your body, maintain. Never let your body-fat percentage drop into the Essential fat range.

Aren't bulking and cutting unhealthy?

Repeatedly and rapidly gaining and losing lots of weight is very unhealthy and therefore not recommended. It plays havoc on your hormones and can have all kinds of other detrimental effects. It is especially unhealthy for women and teenagers.

However, if done correctly, bulking and cutting are not unhealthy. The correct way to bulk and cut, as almost ensured if you follow the steps below, is to take them very slowly and carefully, putting your body into a mild caloric surplus when bulking and into a mild caloric deficit when cutting.

How to bulk and cut: the old way

The old way of bulking and cutting was difficult. It involved:

- manually calculating your total daily energy expenditure (TDEE), which is the number of kilocalories your body needs each day to maintain the same weight
- adding, say, 250 kilocalories if bulking
- subtracting, say, 250 kilocalories if cutting
- deciding on how many of those kilocalories will come from protein, how many will come from fat, and how many will come from carbohydrate (known as your **macronutrient ratio**)
- counting every kilocalorie that you eat and drink with pen and paper, and making sure to meet your daily caloric and macronutrient requirements!

How to bulk and cut: the new way

The new way of bulking and cutting is much easier. Just use an app! I use **MyFitnessPal**. All you have to do is select the relevant app options (see below) depending on whether you want to bulk, cut, or maintain. Then, just:

- use the app to add foods and exercises, and ensure that you meet your daily caloric and macronutrient goals. I explain how to add foods and exercises below, in **How to track your calories and diet**
- every two weeks, enter your new current weight into MyFitnessPal so that it keeps track of your progress and knows how many kilocalories to prescribe.

Note: Whenever you edit your current weight, MyFitnessPal resets your macronutrient ratio settings, so you will have to change them back.

General important notes

Before you start cutting, bulking, or maintaining, take your body-part measurements and body-fat percentage as described in **How to track your progress**, in the **Weight Training Guide**.

Whether bulking, cutting, or maintaining, get the vast majority of your kilocalories from healthy, nutrient-dense foods. MyFitnessPal will tell you what nutrients you're lacking.

If you screw up your diet on occasions — and you surely will! — don't lose enthusiasm and give up; just carry on from where you left off.

You do not need to change your weight training program when bulking, cutting, or maintaining. If necessary, just perform a little more cardio when cutting to assist with fat loss.

There is no perfect way of bulking and cutting that works for everybody. The guidelines below will help you to get started on the right track. However, it's up to you to track your progress and make the necessary adjustments in accordance with your results and preferences.

MyFitnessPal settings for bulking

- Go to the Goals section of MyFitnessPal.
- Enter your Goal Weight. This isn't important. It doesn't affect the app's calculations. Just be realistic.
- For Weekly Goal, select "Gain 0.5 lb per week".
- For Calorie and Macronutrient Goals, set your protein intake to a percentage that ensures that you get 0.59 to 0.82 grams per pound of body weight per day (1.3 to 1.8 grams per kilogram of body weight per day). Set your fat intake to between 20% and 35% based on your own preferences. Set your carbohydrate intake to account for the remaining percentage.

Guidelines for bulking

- Bulk only if your body-fat percentage falls within the Athlete range of Table 6.2.
- If you don't start gaining weight, change your Weekly Goal in MyFitnessPal to "Gain 1 lb per week". This should kick-start your weight gain.
- Bulk for at least six months, preferably longer. You want to allow enough time to build a decent amount of muscle. Remember, you will probably lose a bit of muscle when you cut, and you do not want to lose the small amount that you built and be left exactly where you started!
- If you gain too much weight in the first couple of weeks, don't worry. This is normal if you are new to weight training. It usually occurs because your muscles fill with water and glycogen, which should stop after the first few weeks, leaving your weight to increase at or close to the desired rate. Make sure that the excessive gains aren't all fat by checking your body-fat percentage.
- If you keep gaining too much weight, cut your daily caloric intake in increments of 150 every week until you start gaining the desired amount of weight. You can change your calorie goal in the Goals section of the app.
- Stop bulking if your body-fat percentage exceeds the Fitness range in Table 6.2, and start cutting.

MyFitnessPal settings for cutting

- Go to the Goals section of MyFitnessPal.
- Enter your Goal Weight. As mentioned above, this isn't important. Just be realistic.
- For Weekly Goal, select "Lose 0.5 lb per week".
- For Calorie and Macronutrient Goals, set your protein intake to a percentage that ensures that you get 0.82 to 0.91 grams per pound of body weight per day (1.8 to 2.0 grams per kilogram of body weight per day). If obese, make it per lean body mass instead of per body weight. Set your fat intake to between 20% and 35% based on your own preferences. Set your carbohydrate intake to account for the remaining percentage.

Guidelines for cutting

- If you don't start losing weight, change your weekly goal in MyFitnessPal to "Lose 1 lb per week". This should kick-start your weight loss.
- The cut should be slow and careful to avoid as much muscle loss as possible.
- If you're new to weight training and have a high body-fat percentage, you will probably lose more weight than expected at the start of the cut, which is fine. You can safely lose up to three pounds per week in the first few weeks, after which you should try to lose no more than one pound per week. The reason is that you don't want to end up with ugly, loose skin. What's more, the less fat you have on your body, the more your body will try to burn muscle for energy. To reduce the amount of weight that you're losing, increase your daily caloric intake in increments of 150 every week until you start losing the desired amount. You can change your calorie goal in the Goals section of the app.
- If you stick to your diet, at the end of the week, you can treat yourself to a cheat meal. Yay!

MyFitnessPal settings for maintaining

- Go to the Goals section of MyFitnessPal.

- Enter your Goal Weight, which is the same as your current weight.
- For Weekly Goal, select "Maintain weight".
- For Calorie and Macronutrient Goals, set your protein intake to a percentage that ensures that you get 0.59 to 0.82 grams per pound of body weight per day (1.3 to 1.8 grams per kilogram of body weight per day). Set your fat intake to between 20% and 35% based on your own preferences. Set your carbohydrate intake to account for the remaining percentage.

Guidelines for maintaining

- Maintaining is simply a matter of meeting your daily caloric and macronutrient requirements, tracking your progress, and sticking to your training program.
- As with cutting, you can treat yourself to a cheat meal once a week.
- Note that maintaining with a higher body-fat percentage will give you more potential to keep growing your muscles/curves because you will be able to eat more. The more food you can eat, the more potential your body will have to make gains.

Deciding on how much fat vs carbohydrate

In the above recommendations for protein, fat, and carbohydrate percentages, I suggested that after you select the necessary percentage of protein, you choose a percentage of fat between 20% and 35% based on your own preferences, and that you set your carbohydrate intake to account for the remaining percentage. The following questions will help you to decide how much fat and carbohydrate to select.

- How regularly will you be eating? Fat keeps you satiated for longer than carbohydrate, so if you will be eating only two to three times per day, choose more fat.
- Do you feel exhausted after workouts? If so, make room for more carbohydrate, which is your primary source of energy.
- When bulking, do you find it difficult to eat lots of food every day? If so, choose more fat because fat is more calorie-dense than carbohydrate so you will not have to eat as much food.
- How much do you enjoy fat versus carbohydrate? The less you eat of one, the more you will be able to consume of the other.

When making your decision, keep in mind the importance of getting enough fat-soluble vitamins (A, D, E, and K) and essential fatty acids, and don't forget the crucial role fat plays in the production of testosterone and insulin-like growth factor 1 (IGF-1), which are essential for muscular growth.

How to track your calories and diet

There are quite a few apps out there that make the process of tracking your calories easier. Below, you will learn how to track your calories and diet using probably the most popular app, and the one that I use: **MyFitnessPal**.

The MyFitnessPal app and website

MyFitnessPal is a free app that you can use to track your kilocalories, macronutrients, micronutrients, and exercises. It will help you to make sure that you are eating the right number of kilocalories each day, getting enough of the right vitamins and minerals, and consuming the right quantities of protein, fat, and carbohydrate. The app is available on iOS and Android. If you don't have a smartphone or other mobile device, you can use the MyFitnessPal website (myfitnesspal.com), which offers the same functionalities. After you create an account, you can access it using your login details via the app or website, both of which sync. Of course, the app offers much more convenience than the website. I would buy a smartphone just to use the MyFitnessPal app — that's how helpful it is!

How to use the MyFitnessPal app

A step-by-step explanation of how to use MyFitnessPal is beyond the scope of this chapter. The video on the following page of my website will give you a general outline:

http://weighttraining.guide/nutrition/how-to-track-your-calories-and-diet/

The best way to learn how to use MyFitnessPal is through practice. What follows is just an overview of how to use the app.

Whether you create a MyFitnessPal account on your phone or on the website, during the process, you will be asked for your stats, goals, and activity level.

- Your stats are your height, current weight, gender, and date of birth.
- Your goals are your weekly weight goal (how much weight you want to lose or gain per week, if any) and your ultimate weight goal (what weight you are ultimately aiming for). The options you select will depend on whether you are cutting, maintaining, or bulking.
- Your activity level is the amount of activity you experience in an average day, not including any exercises.

MyFitnessPal then calculates your **net kilocalories**, which is the number of kilocalories you have to eat each day to achieve your goal. All you have to do is add the foods you eat and the exercises you perform to your diary. Periodically, you also have to update your current weight to inform MyFitnessPal of your weight-related progress.

(Note that the way MyFitnessPal calculates your daily caloric requirement is different from the two manual methods of calculating your total daily energy expenditure (TDEE) that I described in **Calories and calorie requirements**. The two manual methods take into account all of your physical activities, including your exercises, and give you your TDEE. As mentioned above, MyFitnessPal does not include your exercises, which you have to add separately. As a result, the net kilocalories figure that it presents will be lower than your TDEE. What's more, when you add an exercise, your net kilocalories figure will go up, meaning that you can eat more food!)

Adding foods to your diary

When you first start using MyFitnessPal, adding foods to your diary takes a bit of time. The process involves searching for the food in the MyFitnessPal database (which contains over 13.6 million entries and still growing), adjusting the quantity of the food to reflect the amount that you ate, and then adding it to your diary. However, the more you use MyFitnessPal, the faster and easier adding foods to your diary becomes, to the point where you should be able to add a whole meal in under a minute. The reason is that the app remembers what you have eaten in the past and makes the process of adding the same foods easier. What's more, you can group foods into meals and recipes, and add the meals and recipes to your diary all in one go. You can even copy meals and recipes from the diaries of other people who have chosen to share their diary with you.

The process of adding foods to your diary is made even easier by the app's barcode scanning feature. If a food has a barcode, just scan it, and MyFitnessPal will locate the food in its database. All you have to do is adjust the quantity before adding it to your diary. If, after a scan, MyFitnessPal doesn't find the right food, you can add the food to the database yourself.

Are the nutritional figures in MyFitnessPal accurate?

Since anybody can add foods to the MyFitnessPal database, some of the entries can be erroneous. Look for a green check mark next to the food, which indicates that the food entry has been checked and approved. Many of the entries without a check mark are also accurate. It's wise to check the nutritional values entered for the foods that you regularly add to your diary.

One figure that is often inaccurate is the food's **sodium** content. Many people enter the food's salt content into the sodium field thinking that they are the same thing. Therefore, keep an eye on that figure.

Keeping an eye on your nutrition

To see how much protein, fat, and carbohydrate you have eaten, as well as how much of each vitamin and dietary mineral you have taken in, visit the Nutrition section of the app. MyFitnessPal breaks it all down for you nicely, and this is what makes the app helpful. After a short while of using MyFitnessPal, you will gain valuable insights into your diet. For example, I discovered that I almost never got enough potassium and that my diet contained way too much fat, even though I thought that my fat intake was low! These insights helped me to make the necessary dietary adjustments. Who knows what you will discover about your diet.

Why don't the fats add up?

MyFitnessPal breaks fat into saturated, monounsaturated, polyunsaturated, and trans fat, as it should do. You may notice that when you add up the figures for these sub-categories of fat, they may not add up to the total amount of fat you have eaten. The reason is that food nutrition labels in many countries, such as the US, are not required to specify the monounsaturated and polyunsaturated fat content of a food, so food companies may only list total fat, saturated fat, and trans fat. This means that if, after you sum the sub-categories, the resultant figure is smaller than the total fat content, you can assume that the remainder is monounsaturated and polyunsaturated fat. Note also that trans fats are monounsaturated and polyunsaturated fats; they do not constitute a separate sub-category of their own.

Adding exercises to your diary

MyFitnessPal lets you add both cardiovascular and strength/weight training exercises to your diary. However, it only calculates how many kilocalories you burned from cardiovascular exercises. In other words, if you add a strength training exercise to your diary via the "Strength Training" button, MyFitnessPal will not try to estimate how many kilocalories you burned, and your net kilocalories figure will not be adjusted. The reason is that estimating the kilocalories burned from strength training is difficult. It depends on too many factors, such as how much weight you lifted, how vigorously you worked out, and how much rest you took between sets. This is a problem because you have to keep track of all of the kilocalories that you eat and burn. The good news is that you can add a strength training workout via the "Cardiovascular" button. Just search for the exercise "Strength training" in the Cardiovascular database, adjust the number of minutes trained, and add the exercise to your diary. The estimate of kilocalories burned will only be a rough estimate, but it's better than nothing. If you tracked how many kilocalories you burned during your workout using a heart rate monitor or other tracking device, you can also add a custom exercise to your personal database.

Upgrading to premium

Upgrading to MyFitnessPal's premium service will give you additional features, such as the ability to set your macronutrient goals in grams instead of percentages and to learn which foods you have eaten rank highest in nutrients that are important to you. The premium service also gets rid of all the ads. However, everything you need is available with the free service.

Weight training supplements

Do you need supplements?

From shakes and bars to pills and powders, there are many different kinds of weight training supplement, some designed to improve performance and others devised to remedy nutritional deficiencies. There are also weight training supplements that promise to help you gain or lose weight. Although you will most likely need a protein supplement to help you to meet your daily protein requirement without exceeding your daily fat requirement, whether or not you need other supplements will depend on your individual circumstances, goals, and preferences.

Always remember, however, that following a nutritious diet, adhering to an effective training program, and ensuring that you get enough rest are the three pillars of weight training success. Supplements cannot compensate for poor diets and ineffective training regimens. Before you think about supplements, you should focus on learning and implementing proper nutrition and exercise. Only after you have maximized your results by implementing proper nutrition and exercise should you consider supplementation.

Can weight training supplements be dangerous?

Be careful of weight training supplements. They are often not regulated, which means that there is no guarantee that the product will contain what it says on the tin. There's also the risk that the product is contaminated with banned or illegal substances, such as steroids, stimulants, and hormones. What's more, many weight training supplements that you buy are imitations. Take a brief glance at the reviews of some protein powders on Amazon.com and you will likely see customers complaining about receiving an imitation item! That's why the packaging of many legitimate products, such as protein powders, includes a hologram, which makes counterfeiting more difficult. Therefore, if you are going to buy a supplement, make sure that it is legitimate, legal, and safe.

Types of supplement

Whey and casein protein powders

One of the weight training supplements that you will almost certainly need is a protein powder. Protein powders are convenient, cost-effective, and great for before and after a workout. They are very useful in helping you to reach your daily protein requirement without consuming too much fat. The powders can be used to make shakes or anything in which they can be dissolved, including bars, cakes, and other bakes. The most popular varieties of protein powder are **whey** and **casein**, with whey being the most popular.

Whey is derived from milk, and is a by-product of cheese production. It is digested quickly by the body and provides a balanced source of all nine essential amino acids, including the branched-chain amino acids leucine, isoleucine, and valine.

Casein also comes from milk and provides all nine essential amino acids, including the branched-chain amino acids leucine, isoleucine, and valine. However, it contains less leucine than whey does and is digested slowly by the body. The reason is that casein forms a gel in the stomach, which provides a slow and sustained release of amino acids into the bloodstream.

The rate of a protein's digestion is important for muscle protein balance. Because whey is digested quickly, it causes a rapid increase in blood amino acids and protein synthesis. However, it is short-lived, which can open the room for protein breakdown. Casein, on the other hand, causes a slow but prolonged increase in blood amino acids, which can be better at preventing muscle protein breakdown.

Since whey provides a quick burst of amino acids and casein provides a more prolonged source of amino acids, they can be used alone or in combination to exploit their unique characteristics. For example, use casein powder to make bedtime shakes because it promotes a sustained anti-catabolic environment, and use whey powder when you need a quick surge of amino acids, such as before and after a workout, and first thing in the morning. Mix whey in a large glass of milk to get the added benefit of naturally occurring casein.

Creatine, the performance enhancer

Creatine is a protein that enhances your muscles' ability to perform. It is naturally synthesized in your body and can also be found in protein-rich foods, such as red meat and fish. After being eaten, creatine is used to make **creatine phosphate** (also known as **phosphocreatine**), which is used to synthesize **adenosine triphosphate** (**ATP**), the compound in which all of the cells in your body store and use energy. Boosting muscle creatine phosphate levels increases your strength and endurance, and allows you to recover faster between exertions. The more creatine phosphate there is in your muscle cells, the more fuel the cells will have to work, the harder you will be able to train, and the more you will stimulate growth in muscles or curves. Creatine has also been found to increase bone mineral density, improve glucose metabolism, and enhance brain performance — making it the supplement of choice for many athletes and one of the most popular weight training supplements in the bodybuilding industry.

Creatine is permitted by the International Olympic Committee, as well as professional sports and the National Collegiate Athletic Association (NCAA). However, the NCAA no longer allows colleges to supply creatine to their students with school funds.

Tribulus terrestris, the "testosterone booster"

Also known as the **puncture vine**, *Tribulus terrestris* is a Mediterranean plant that is presented as a natural alternative to anabolic steroids. Mostly recommended for male virility, it was popularized by IFBB bodybuilding champion Jeffrey Petermann in the early 1970s as a supplement that can boost the body's natural testosterone levels, thus improving male sexual performance and helping to build muscle. However, while *Tribulus terrestris* does seem to have libido-enhancing properties (especially in rats), scientific studies have failed to find evidence for the claim that it can boost testosterone levels in humans. In fact, there is no evidence that *Tribulus terrestris* can enhance sports performance or increase muscular growth in any way. I mention it here only to dissuade you from ever trying it.

Ephedrine, the banned fat burner

Ephedrine is a central nervous system stimulant derived from the ephedra (or Ma-huang) plant. In its herbal form, it has been used for over 2,000 years by the Chinese to treat asthma, nasal congestion, and allergies. Resembling adrenaline, ephedrine increases basal metabolic rate (BMR), thus spurring the body to burn calories faster. However, the dietary supplement was banned by the FDA in 2004 because it was found to be unsafe and presents little proven benefit.

Weight gainers

Some individuals, commonly known as **"hard gainers"**, have a very fast metabolism, making gaining weight and muscle very difficult. Weight gainers are supplements designed to help hard gainers to increase body mass by boosting caloric intake. The supplements are packed with kilocalories, usually delivered in the form of a combination of proteins (usually whey and casein) and both low-glycemic and high-glycemic carbohydrates. The supplements may also include omega-3 fatty acids and fiber.

Weight gainers are of course also very useful when you are bulking. They can help you to boost your caloric intake without having to spend all day in the fridge. A single shake can provide a whole meal's worth or more of kilocalories!

Nutrient timing

For weight training success, nutrient timing is important. Nutrient timing is the study of delivering the right combinations of the right nutrients at the right times to your body to ensure the best possible results. Two meals are especially important for your progress: your **pre-workout meal** and your **post-workout meal**. Eating the right foods at the right times both before and after your workout will provide your body with what it needs to achieve optimal exercise performance, recovery, and growth.

Pre-workout nutrition

Eating before you exercise may sometimes not be necessary. Whether or not you need a pre-workout meal depends on when you last ate, and whether or not you ate enough protein. If it has been several hours since you last ate, eating some fast-digesting protein (for example, whey) an hour or so before you hit the gym will help to increase muscle protein synthesis, and consuming some carbohydrate with that protein will give you the energy you need for an effective workout. The pre-workout carbohydrate will also help you to maintain blood sugar levels, delay the fatigue of your muscles, improve your endurance, and spare the glycogen in your muscle tissues. This is important because when muscle glycogen levels are low, exercise-induced muscle breakdown can be accelerated. High-glycemic carbohydrates are best for short (one-hour), high-intensity workouts, whereas low-glycemic carbohydrates are preferred for long (two-hour or more), endurance workouts.

Post-workout nutrition

It is well known that consuming a protein-rich meal after a workout can improve your muscle-building results. It does this by minimizing post-workout muscle protein breakdown and maximizing protein synthesis. One study suggests that 20 grams of easy-to-digest protein is the optimal amount for muscle growth immediately after exercise. When athletes consumed less than 20 grams, they gained less muscle; when they consumed more than 25 grams, they experienced no further muscle gains. Note, however, that the athletes weighed around 85 kilograms (187 pounds). If you weigh significantly more than this, you will need a bit more protein, and if you weigh significantly less, you will need a bit less protein.

For best results, the post-workout meal should also include carbohydrate, with the amount of carbohydrate usually recommended being 1.0 gram per kilogram of body weight (0.45 grams per pound of body weight). The reason that carbohydrate should be consumed with the protein is that it promotes a greater release of insulin, which facilitates the transport of glucose and amino acids into muscle cells. The more insulin there is available, the more glucose and amino acids can be carried into muscles for protein synthesis. Insulin also reduces the stress hormone cortisol, which is known to suppress protein synthesis, stimulate protein breakdown, and even affect testosterone production.

Another reason to eat carbohydrate after a workout is to replenish muscle glycogen stores. As explained above, maintaining muscle glycogen stores reduces the need for muscle protein breakdown.

PART 3: WEIGHT TRAINING PROGRAMS

Chapter 7: Men's weight training programs

Overview of men's training programs

Programs for men

As summarized in Table 7.1, there are three weight training programs for men.

Program	Mesocycle	Duration (weeks)	Workouts Per Week	Workout duration (mins)	Repeatable?
Muscle and Strength	Beginner	12	3-5	30–40	No
	Muscle	6	5	45–50	Yes
	Muscle 2	8	4	45–50	Yes
	Muscle and Strength	12	4	45–50 (longer on strength days)	Yes
	Muscle and Strength 2	9	5	45–50 (longer on strength days)	Yes
	Muscle and Strength 3	12	4	40–45 (longer on strength days)	Yes
Men's Plateau Buster	N/A	9	5	55–60 (longer on strength days)	Yes
Minimalistic Program for Busy Men	N/A	12	4	25–30	Yes

Table 7.1. Summary of the three weight training programs for men, including each program's duration, number of workouts per week, approximate workout duration, and whether or not the program can be repeated. The workout duration does not include the warmup and cooldown.

The first program, **Muscle and Strength**, actually consists of six smaller programs (mesocycles). As its name implies, Muscle and Strength is intended for men who want to develop maximum muscle and strength.

The **Men's Plateau Buster** is a stand-alone program that you can use if you ever experience a plateau (a plateau is when you stop making progress due to your body becoming adapted to the training stimulus). Since the program is designed to produce the same results as Muscle and Strength, you can also include it as part of Muscle and Strength and use it after Muscle and Strength 3.

The **Minimalistic Program for Busy Men** is another stand-alone program. It is designed to provide a quick and effective full-body workout for men who have very little time to spare for the gym.

You can complete the training programs at any gym or at home using the alternative exercises that I have provided for each program and the following equipment:

- Adjustable bench
- Dumbbells
- Pull-up bar
- Barbell
- Power rack for safety
- Clip resistance bands (optional but important in the absence of a cable machine and leg-curling machine)
- Ankle straps (optional but important for leg curls in the absence of a leg-curling machine)
- Ab wheel (optional)
- Dip bars (optional)

All of the programs and the way they were designed will be explored in detail below.

General instructions

If a beginner, you should start from the beginner program, after which you can move on to either the Muscle and Strength programs or the minimalistic program, depending on your preferences.

If experienced, you can start from any program that you choose as long as you meet the suitability criteria (see tables 7.2 and 7.3).

Muscle and Strength

Muscle and Strength is a comprehensive long-term weight training program that was meticulously designed to:

- build and maintain major muscle mass and strength
- strengthen your core, which is important for stability, body-wide strength, power generation, and power transfer
- strengthen your body's primal movement patterns, which is important for functional strength, balance, coordination, athleticism, and performance
- encourage the right strength balances between your opposing muscle groups, which is important for proper posture and movement, and to prevent imbalance-related injuries.

The program does this by using, or adhering to, a combination of:

- major mass-building compound exercises
- functional exercises

- undulating periodization
- intensity training techniques
- recommended muscle strength balance ratios.

In programming terminology, the long-term Muscle and Strength program is a **macrocycle** ("big cycle"). The six individual programs that make up Muscle and Strength (from the Men's Beginner Program to Muscle and Strength 3) are known as **mesocycles** ("middle cycles"). Although not expressed in Table 7.1, most of the mesocycles are themselves divided into **microcycles** ("small cycles"). The mesocycles and microcycles incorporate variations in training, which will be explained in the mesocycle overview.

Muscle and Strength lasts for a minimum of one year and 12 weeks if you move from mesocycle to mesocycle and take a deload week after each one. A deload week is a week during which you either rest or train lightly. However, apart from the beginner mesocycle, you do not have to move from one mesocycle straight on to the next one. I balanced the exercises in each mesocycle as best as I could so that you can keep repeating each mesocycle over and over without much of a risk of developing muscular imbalances. As such, you can repeat each mesocycle as many times as you want to before moving on to the next one. This will ensure that you get the most out of each mesocycle and the macrocycle as a whole.

In fact, you don't have to move on at all. If you enjoy a particular mesocycle, you can stick to it. Provided you keep increasing the amount of weight that you lift, as requested in the instructions of each mesocycle, you should see continual progress for a significant amount of time. Just make sure that you take a deload week before repeating a mesocycle or moving on to the next mesocycle.

Note that the deload weeks are important. Please do not ignore them. They will help you to fully recover and therefore keep making progress. They will also increase your likelihood of not giving up.

Mesocycle overview

Men's Beginner

Before I provide an overview of each mesocycle (Table 7.2), I remind you that training in different rep ranges leads to the development of different muscle properties. More specifically, using a weight with which you can perform 13–20 reps in good form is optimal for developing muscular endurance; using a weight with which you can only perform 6–12 reps in good form (i.e. a heavy weight) is optimal for developing muscular size; and using a weight with which you can only perform 2–6 reps in good form (i.e. a very heavy weight) is optimal for developing muscular strength.

Focusing mostly on the 13+ rep range, the 12-week Men's Beginner mesocycle is designed to build a strong foundation of muscular endurance upon which muscular size and strength can be built in the more advanced mesocycles. It is intended for beginners, lifters who have less than three months of consistent weight training experience, and experienced lifters who haven't trained for over three months.

116

Mesocycle	Rep ranges	Intensity technique	Experience required (months)
Men's Beginner	13+	None	None
Muscle	9–11	Supersets	3
Muscle 2	9–11, 6–8	Training to failure	6
Muscle and Strength	9–11, 6–8, 3–5	Dropsets	9
Muscle and Strength 2	9–11, 6–8, 3–5	Rest–pause sets	12
Muscle and Strength 3	9–11, 6–8, 3–5	Supersets	12

Table 7.2. The rep ranges and intensity techniques of each mesocycle, along with the level of experience required to start from the mesocycle.

Muscle

The 6-week Muscle mesocycle starts to build muscular size, as derived from the 9–11 rep range. It also incorporates an intensity technique known as **superset training**. You can start from this mesocycle without having to go through the Men's Beginner mesocycle only if you have at least three months of consistent weight training experience.

Muscle 2

The 8-week Muscle 2 mesocycle is composed of microcycles that alternate between the 9–11 and 6–8 rep ranges. While both rep ranges are for developing muscular size, the 6–8 rep range helps to develop more strength. This mesocycle includes an intensity technique known as **training to failure**. You can start from this mesocycle only if you have at least six months of consistent training experience.

Muscle and Strength

The 12-week Muscle and Strength mesocycle consists of microcycles that alternate between the 9–11, 6–8, and 3–5 rep ranges. The first two rep ranges are for building muscle; the last rep range is for developing muscular strength. The mesocycle also includes an intensity technique called **dropset training**. You can start from this mesocycle only if you have at least nine months of consistent weight training experience.

Muscle and Strength 2

Like the Muscle and Strength mesocycle, the 9-week Muscle and Strength 2 mesocycle consists of microcycles that alternate between the 9–11, 6–8, and 3–5 rep ranges for developing both muscular size and strength. It includes an intensity training technique known as **rest–pause training**. You can start from this mesocycle only if you have at least 12 months of consistent training experience.

Muscle and Strength 3

Although the 12-week Muscle and Strength 3 mesocycle also comprises microcycles that alternate between the 9–11, 6–8, and 3–5 rep ranges, it is different from the other mesocycles in that all of the exercises are arranged into supersets. As such, the workouts are more intense and quicker to complete. You can start from this mesocycle only if you have at least 12 months of consistent weight training experience.

Why alternate between rep ranges?

Most weight training programs that you have come across have probably followed either no progression or a linear progression through rep ranges, beginning with 13–20 (for muscular endurance), moving on to 6–12 (for muscular size), and maybe ending with 2–6 (for muscular strength). This arrangement is known as **linear periodization**. The problem with linear periodization is that when you move from one rep range to another, you start to lose the properties that you developed in the previous rep range. My programs are based on an arrangement called **undulating periodization**, wherein the rep ranges are maintained as you progress and alternated in microcycles. This ensures that as you progress, the properties that you developed in previous mesocycles (endurance, size, or strength) are not only maintained but also continually developed while you also develop new properties. Note that only the size and strength rep ranges are maintained, not the endurance rep range.

Overview of the other training programs for men

Men's Plateau Buster

The 9-week Men's Plateau Buster is your weapon for breaking out of plateaus, should they ever occur. You can also use it as if it's the seventh Muscle and Strength mesocycle, and repeat it as many times as you want to.

As with the advanced Muscle and Strength mesocycles, the Men's Plateau Buster consists of microcycles that alternate between the 9–11, 6–8, and 3–5 rep ranges (Table 7.3). The difference is that most of the exercises are arranged in accordance with an advanced intensity protocol known as **pre-exhaustion training**, which will ensure that you partially exhaust prime mover muscles using isolation exercises before you move on to the main compound exercises. Pre-exhaustion of prime movers makes them work much harder during the compound exercises, thus amplifying the stimulus for development and increasing your chances of kick-starting stunted progress.

If you're new to weight training and follow the Muscle and Strength program, you will almost certainly not need this program as a plateau buster for at least a couple of years. However, if you ever do need it, it should ensure that you never stop making progress.

Program	Rep ranges	Intensity technique	Experience required
Men's Plateau Buster	9–11, 6–8, 3–5	Pre-exhaustion	12 months
Minimalistic Program for Busy Men	9–11, 6–8	Supersets	Completion of microcycles 1–3 of the Men's Beginner mesocycle

Table 7.3. The rep ranges and intensity techniques of the men's plateau buster and minimalistic programs, along with the level of experience required to start from each program.

Minimalistic Program for Busy Men

The 12-week Minimalistic Program for Busy Men is for you if you don't have much time for workouts. Alternating between the 9–11 and 6–8 rep ranges, the workouts include the bare minimum of exercises and sets necessary to get an effective full-body workout. What's more, the exercises are arranged into supersets, which means that you can fly through them very rapidly.

You can repeat the Minimalistic Program for Busy Men as many times as you want to. If a beginner, ideally, before you start the program, you should have completed at least microcycles 1 through 3 of the Men's Beginner mesocycle. As with the minimalistic workouts, the workouts of microcycles 1 through 3 of the Men's Beginner mesocycle are short, and they will help you to develop a small foundation of muscular endurance upon which the Minimalistic Program for Busy Men can build.

How the programs were designed

Exercise selection

The purpose of all of the training programs for men is to build and maintain muscular mass and strength, strengthen the core, strengthen the body's primal movement patterns, and encourage the right strength balances between opposing muscle groups. Most of the exercises were selected to fulfil those objectives. However, some exercises were included to serve other purposes, such as to prepare you in one mesocycle to move on to more advanced exercises in the following mesocycle, or simply to add variation to the workouts to keep you engaged.

Exercises for maximum muscle and strength

To maximize gains in muscle and strength, I ensured that the programs are dominated by major compound exercises (for example, the barbell squat). Compound exercises simultaneously target multiple muscles and involve the movement of two or more joints (or pairs of joints). They are different from isolation exercises (for example, the dumbbell curl), which target fewer muscles (sometimes only one) and involve the movement of only one joint (or one pair of joints). Focusing on major compound exercises ensures that you:

- stimulate simultaneous growth in the maximum number of muscles
- flood your body with testosterone and human growth hormone, which will boost the development of muscle and strength throughout your entire body
- strengthen your base and core, which will help you to lift even more weight and thus feed the cycle of growth.

All of this will ensure that you pack on the most amount of muscle and strength, and get maximum results in the least amount of time.

Another benefit of compound exercises is that their movements are more natural than the movements of isolation exercises, which means that they are much better at improving your functional strength, balance, coordination, athleticism, and performance. What's more, compound exercises provide a better cardiovascular workout.

Exercises to strengthen primal movement patterns

Functional strength is the kind of strength that is useful outside of the gym, in everyday activities. You develop functional strength by strengthening the ways in which your body is designed to move.

The ways in which your body is designed to move can be broken down into seven "primal" movement patterns:

1. Squatting
2. Lunging (forward, sideways, or backward)
3. Flexing/Extending the hips
4. Pushing (horizontally or vertically)
5. Pulling (horizontally or vertically)
6. Twisting (or resisting twisting forces)
7. Walking/Running (gait)

You use these primal movement patterns in various combinations every day of your life. By strengthening them, you not only develop a functionally strong body but also:

- enhance your motor control, coordination, balance, and flexibility
- become more equipped for everyday activities
- improve your overall fitness, athleticism, and performance.

Unfortunately, most training programs that you encounter do not cover these movement patterns. Instead, they focus on training muscles, often in isolation, which is not how the body is designed to work. Rest assured that the weight training programs in this book, together with the FCT cardio program, incorporate effective functional training and give you the benefits outlined above.

Exercises to strengthen your core

An important element of having a functionally strong body is to have a strong core. Your core isn't just your rectus abdominis and lower back; it's your entire torso, especially all of the deep muscles that attach to your spinal column and pelvis. Your core muscles help to:

- stabilize your body when you lift
- transfer weight from one side of your body to the other
- transfer weight from your lower body to your upper body.

Your core is also where you generate much of your power. As such, it acts as your power base, power transfer center, and stabilization facility. Having a strong core is therefore of major importance for progress and overall fitness and athleticism.

Proper core training involves performing a range of major compound and functional exercises designed to strengthen both the deep and superficial muscles of the core, ideally, both dynamically and isometrically. All of the weight training programs in this book incorporate effective dynamic core training, while some also include isometric core training.

Exercise balance

When training, it's important to develop a balanced musculature. Ideally, the strengths of opposing muscle groups, the strength of the right side of your body compared with the left side, and the strength of your upper body compared with your lower body should adhere to recommended muscle strength balance ratios. The reason is that if opposing regions of your body or opposing muscle groups develop significant differences in strength, performance can be jeopardized, and the risk of sustaining injuries and developing problems related to muscle tightness, joint instability, posture, and gait can be increased.

Athletes prevent or fix imbalances by approaching a personal trainer, who identifies the strength ratios of their muscles using one-repetition maximum testing and then prescribes a training program to fix any imbalances or ensure that imbalances are not developed. The least you can do as a gym-goer and fitness enthusiast who cares about his physique is follow weight training programs that are balanced and therefore reduce your likelihood of developing imbalances. In order to reduce your likelihood of developing imbalances while using the programs in this book, I designed them in accordance with the muscle strength balance ratios recommended by the International Fitness Professionals Association (IFPA; Table 7.4).

Muscle group	Muscle balance ratio
Hip flexors and extensors	1:1
Knee flexors and extensors	2:3
Shoulder flexors and extensors	2:3

Shoulder internal and external rotators	3:2
Elbow flexors and extensors	1:1
Trunk flexors and extensors	1:1
Ankle plantar flexors and dorsiflexors	3:1

Table 7.4. Muscle strength balance ratios recommended by the IFPA.

The strategy that I used was to:

- make note of the target and synergistic muscles of each exercise, as revealed on ExRx.net
- ensure that the number of exercises and sets for opposing muscles and opposing movement patterns generally agree with the above ratios.

For example, since you should be able to lift the same amount of weight with your elbow flexors as with your elbow extensors, I have tried to make sure that the number of exercises and sets that hit those muscles is approximately equal.

Note that balancing the Men's Beginner program wasn't as important as balancing the other programs because the Men's Beginner program isn't intended to be repeated over and over again and is designed to prepare you for the subsequent programs. Even so, it is still relatively balanced.

Summary of programming rules and objectives

When designing the training programs for men, I tried to follow or satisfy the following rules and objectives:

- Train all muscle groups at least twice a week
- Strengthen all primal movement patterns using compound and functional exercises
- Prescribe exercises and sets for opposing muscles and movement patterns in accordance with recommended muscle strength balance ratios
- Undulate rep ranges to simultaneously develop multiple muscle properties and maintain properties developed in previous mesocycles
- Strengthen the core using compound, functional, and unilateral exercises
- Train the core dynamically and isometrically
- Only include exercises the equipment for which should be available in any gym
- Incorporate exercise variation to maintain engagement
- Avoid exercises that have a high risk-to-benefit ratio, such as the close-grip upright row and behind-the-neck pulls and presses
- Generally favor free-weight exercises over machine exercises
- Avoid overworking of the supraspinatus muscle, which is a common mistake
- Train large muscle groups before small muscle groups

- Prescribe more sets for large muscle groups than for small muscle groups
- If a muscle has multiple heads, include exercises that emphasize each head
- Train large heads of individual muscles before small heads
- Keep workouts to approximately 18 sets (the more advanced workouts include up to 21 sets)
- Force gradual but definite progress from mesocycle to mesocycle
- Ensure adequate rest by enforcing regular deload weeks

Alternative exercises

If you get bored of an exercise, or if you can't perform one of the exercises for some reason, I have provided suitable alternatives below that maintain a similar balance.

Legs and glutes

- Hyperextension – Straight-leg deadlift
- Romanian deadlift – Cable pull-through
- Squat – Front squat – Hack squat – Sumo squat – Zercher squat – Jefferson squat
- Forward/Rear/Side lunge – Step-up – Split squat –Bulgarian split squat
- Lying leg curl – Seated leg curl – Inverse leg curl
- Machine standing calf raise – Standing one-leg dumbbell calf raise – Leg-press calf press
- Barbell hip thrust – Barbell glute bridge

Back

- Lat pull-down – Pull-up (medium grip is best)
- Close neutral grip lat pull-down – Underhand lat pull-down – Chin-up
- Bent-over dumbbell row – Barbell row – T-bar row – Inverted row – Straight-back seated cable row

Chest

- Bench press – Push-up – Cable/Machine chest press
- Incline reverse-grip bench press – Incline bench press – Incline push-up – Pike push-up
- Low cable cross-over – Incline dumbbell fly

Shoulders

- Overhead press – Arnold press
- Cable face pull – Dumbbell face pull – Cuban rotation
- Lying dumbbell external shoulder rotation – Cable external shoulder rotation

Arms

- Triceps rope push-down – Dumbbell/Cable kickback – Triceps overhead extension – Lying triceps extension (French press) – Skull crusher
- Triceps dip – Bench dip – Diamond push-up – Close-grip bench press/push-up
- Dumbbell/Barbell curl – EZ bar curl (bar must have minimal camber)

- Preacher curl – Concentration curl
- Hammer curl – Reverse curl

Core

- Front plank – Ab walkout – Inch worm – Wheel rollout
- Cable wood chop – Weighted Russian twist – Weighted lying oblique twist
- Lying leg raise – Hanging leg raise – Captain's chair leg raise
- Lying straight leg raise – Hanging straight leg raise – Captain's chair straight leg raise
- Lying leg and hip raise – Hanging leg and hip raise – Captain's chair leg and hip raise

Men's Beginner

Description

The 12-week Men's Beginner program is designed to:

- introduce your body to physical exercise
- introduce you to a variety of exercises, training equipment, and training splits
- train all of your major muscle groups
- strengthen your core and primal movement patterns
- encourage body-wide neuromuscular adaptation
- develop a strong foundation of muscular endurance.

The Men's Beginner program is very important because it will lay a strong foundation upon which you can safely build in the subsequent programs. Without this strong foundation, you will be at risk of injury. By the end of the program, you should have developed significant strength (mostly due to neuromuscular adaptation), muscular endurance, and muscular tone, as well as dramatically improved your overall fitness.

The program is divided into four microcycles, each one lasting for three weeks. The first two microcycles focus on full-body circuit training, which means that you will be training your entire body in each workout and having minimal rest between exercises. The last two microcycles focus on split training, which means that you will be dividing your body and training different parts in different workouts.

Please don't be intimidated by the number of exercises in some of the workouts. You will be flying through them with very little rest, so the workouts will be over very quickly.

Please read the **Overview of men's training programs**, at the beginning of this chapter, before you start this program.

Suitability

- Beginners
- Lifters with less than 3 months of consistent weight training experience
- Experienced lifters who haven't trained for more than 3 months

General instructions

- Always use an amount of weight that makes completing the reps challenging.
- Whenever you have to increase the weight, add a maximum of 5 lb (2.5 kg) to upper-body exercises or 10 lb (5 kg) to lower-body exercises — just enough to make the rep range challenging again.
- Complete the exercises in the order provided.
- Try to master the proper form of each exercise, including proper breathing technique. Instructions for most exercises are available on my website, **weighttraining.guide**. Also, try to develop a mental connection with your muscles and the movement patterns.
- If training at home in the absence of cable machines and other specialized equipment, see below the exercise tables for exercise alternatives.
- Don't forget to warm up before, and cool down after, each workout.
- Once you have completed the Men's Beginner program, you must take a deload week (a week during which you must either rest or train lightly). Only then can you move on to the next program.

Specific instructions for each microcycle are presented below.

Microcycle 1: Full-body circuit (3 weeks)

- For microcycle 1, you will perform a full-body circuit.
- Complete 2 circuits per workout.
- Complete 3 workouts per week, with at least 1 day of rest between each workout (i.e. AXAXAXX, where "A" is a workout day and "X" is a rest day).
- Rest for only 20 to 30 seconds between exercises.
- Rest for 2 to 3 minutes between the circuits.
- Each workout should take less than 30 minutes.

Exercise	Reps
Dumbbell squat*	15–18
Wide-grip lat pull-down	15–18
Seated or lying leg curl	15–18
Dumbbell bench press	15–18
Machine standing calf raise	25–30

Seated cable row	15–18
Bicycle crunch	15–20
Seated dumbbell overhead press	15–18
Dumbbell curl	15–18
Dumbbell kickback	15–18
*Bodyweight squat for first week	

Alternatives for cable/machine exercises

- Wide-grip lat pull-down — Wide-grip band lat pull-down or wide-grip self-assisted pull-up
- Seated or lying leg curl — Inverse leg curl, stability ball leg curl, or band leg curl
- Machine standing calf raise — Standing dumbbell one-leg calf raise or band standing calf raise
- Seated cable row — Bent-over dumbbell row, bent-over barbell row, or band row

Microcycle 2: Full-body circuit (3 weeks)

- For microcycle 2, you will perform another full-body circuit.
- Complete either 3 workouts a week (AXAXAXX) or a workout every other day (AX).
- Complete 2 circuits per workout.
- Rest for only 20 to 30 seconds between exercises.
- Rest for 2 to 3 minutes before starting the second circuit.
- Each workout should take less than 35 minutes.

Exercise	Reps
Barbell squat	13–15
Close neutral grip lat pull-down	13–15
Dumbbell Romanian deadlift	13–15
Push-up (on knees if necessary)	13–15
Dumbbell lunge	13–15
Bent-over dumbbell row	13–15
Seated or lying leg curl	13–15
Dumbbell one-arm overhead press	13–15

Standing dumbbell one-leg calf raise	25–30
Bicycle crunch	20–25
EZ bar curl	13–15

Alternatives for cable/machine exercises

- Close neutral grip lat pull-down — Close neutral grip band lat pull-down or close neutral grip self-assisted pull-up
- Seated or lying leg curl — Inverse leg curl, stability ball leg curl, or band leg curl

Microcycle 3: Upper–Lower split (3 weeks)

- For microcycle 3, you will perform an upper–lower split. This means that you will train all of your upper body in one workout (Workout A) and all of your lower body in another workout (Workout B). Also, instead of circuit training, you will perform set training, which means that you will complete all of the sets for one exercise before moving on to the sets of the following exercise.
- The recommended workout schedules are ABXABXX or ABX.
- Rest for only 20 to 30 seconds between sets.
- Rest for only 60 to 90 seconds between exercises.
- Each workout should take less than 40 minutes.

Workout A (Upper body)	
Exercise	**Sets x Reps**
One-arm lat pull-down	2 x 13–15
Seated cable row	2 x 13–15
Barbell bench press	2 x 13–15
Barbell overhead press	2 x 13–15
Cable face pull	2 x 13–15
Triceps rope push-down	2 x 13–15
Dumbbell concentration curl	2 x 13–15
Cable twist	2 x 13–15
Front plank	2 x 45–60 s
s = seconds	

Workout B (Lower body)	
Exercise	Sets x Reps
Barbell front squat	2 x 13–15
Dumbbell rear lunge	2 x 13–15
Barbell Romanian deadlift	2 x 13–15
Seated or lying leg curl	2 x 13–15
Standing dumbbell one-leg calf raise	2 x 20–25
Machine seated calf raise	2 x 20–25
Lying side hip raise	2 x 20–25
Bicycle crunch	2 x 20–25
Lying leg and hip raise	2 x 15–20

Alternatives for cable/machine exercises

- One-arm lat pull-down — One-arm band lat pull-down or self-assisted pull-up
- Seated cable row — Bent-over dumbbell row, bent-over barbell row, or band row
- Cable face pull — Dumbbell face pull or band face pull
- Triceps rope push-down — Dumbbell kickback or triceps band push-down
- Cable twist — Weighted Russian twist or band twist
- Seated or lying leg curl — Inverse leg curl, one-leg stability ball leg curl, or band leg curl
- Machine seated calf raise — Barbell seated calf raise

Microcycle 4: 3-day split (3 weeks)

- For microcycle 4, you will perform a 3-day split in which you will train your back, biceps, and core in Workout A; your chest, shoulders, triceps, and core in Workout B; and your legs and core in Workout C.
- The recommended workout schedules are ABCXABX (then start from C the next week) or ABCX (i.e. three days on, one day off).
- Rest for only 20 to 30 seconds between sets.
- Rest for only 60 to 90 seconds between exercises.
- Each workout should take less than 35 minutes.

Workout A (Back, biceps, core)	
Exercise	**Sets x Reps**
Barbell sumo deadlift	2 x 12–14
Medium-grip lat pull-down	2 x 12–14
Cable twisting one-arm row	2 x 12–14
Dumbbell curl	2 x 12–14
Barbell reverse curl	2 x 12–14
Lying side hip raise	2 x 25–30
Bicycle crunch	2 x 25–30
Seated leg raise	2 x 25–30

Workout B (Chest, shoulders, triceps, core)	
Exercise	**Sets x Reps**
Barbell bench press	2 x 12–14
Inline reverse-grip dumbbell bench press	2 x 12–14
Dumbbell one-arm overhead press	2 x 12–14
Dumbbell bent-over lateral raise	2 x 12–14
Cable face pull	2 x 12–14
Diamond push-up (on knees if necessary)	2 x 12–14
Decline dumbbell triceps extension	2 x 12–14
Captain's chair leg and hip raise	2 x 12–14

Workout C (Legs and core)	
Exercise	**Sets x Reps**
Barbell sumo squat	2 x 12–14
Dumbbell side lunge	2 x 12–14
Weighted one-leg hip thrust	2 x 12–14
Seated or lying leg curl	2 x 12–14

Machine standing calf raise	2 x 20–25
Machine seated calf raise	2 x 20–25
Wheel rollout	2 x 10–15
Cable wood chop	2 x 12–14

Alternatives for cable/machine exercises

- Medium-grip lat pull-down — Medium-grip band lat pull-down or medium-grip self-assisted pull-up
- Cable twisting one-arm row — Band twisting one-arm row or dumbbell twisting row
- Cable face pull — Band face pull or dumbbell face pull
- Captain's chair leg and hip raise — Lying or hanging leg and hip raise
- Seated or lying leg curl — Inverse leg curl, one-leg stability ball leg curl, or band leg curl
- Machine standing calf raise — Standing dumbbell one-leg calf raise or band standing calf raise
- Machine seated calf raise — Barbell seated calf raise
- Wheel rollout — Ab walkout or inch worm
- Cable wood chop — Band wood chop or weighted Russian twist

Muscle

Description

The 6-week Muscle program is designed to:

- train all of your major muscle groups
- build muscle in the 9–11 rep range
- strengthen your core and primal movement patterns
- introduce you to the intensity technique of superset training.

The program is a 3-day training split, which means that you will divide your body into three and train each of the three sections in a separate workout. In Workout A, you will train your back, biceps, and core; in Workout B, you will train your chest, shoulders, triceps, and core; and in Workout C, you will train your legs and core.

Please read the **Overview of men's training programs**, at the beginning of this chapter, before you start this program.

Suitability

- Lifters who have completed the Men's Beginner program
- Anyone who has at least 3 months of consistent weight training experience

Instructions

- Complete the workouts (A, B, and C) in the order provided.
- The recommend workout schedules are ABCX (i.e. three days on, one day off) or ABCXABX (three days on, one day off, two days on, one day off, then carry on from where you left off).
- Perform the exercises in the order provided.
- Complete all of the sets for each exercise before moving on to the sets of the next exercise.
- Rest for 30–90 seconds between the sets.
- Rest for 1–2 minutes between the exercises.
- Always use an amount of weight that will make completing the reps challenging.
- Whenever you have to increase the weight, add a maximum of 5 lb (2.5 kg) to upper-body exercises or 10 lb (5 kg) to lower-body exercises.
- Try to master the proper form of each exercise, including proper breathing technique. Instructions for most exercises are available on my website, **weighttraining.guide**. Also, try to develop a mental connection with your muscles and with the movement patterns as you train.
- If you get bored of an exercise, see the **Overview of men's training programs** for alternatives.
- If training at home in the absence of cable machines and other specialized equipment, see below the exercise tables for exercise alternatives.
- The exercises marked with an asterisk (*) are to be performed as a superset if possible, which means that after you perform a set of one exercise, you must perform a set of the other exercise without resting.
- Don't forget to warm up before, and cool down after, each workout.
- Once you have completed the Muscle program, you must take a deload week. Only then can you move on to the next program or redo the same program.

Workout A (Back, biceps, core)	
Exercise	**Sets x Reps**
Barbell deadlift	3 x 9–11
Pull-up with dumbbell between feet	3 x 9–11
Seated cable row	2 x 9–11
Bent-over dumbbell row	2 x 9–11
EZ bar curl*	3 x 9–11
Wheel rollout*	3 x 10–15

Dumbbell lying external shoulder rotation	2 x 15–20
*To be performed as a superset	

Workout B (Chest, shoulders, triceps, core)	
Exercise	Sets x Reps
Barbell bench press	3 x 9–11
Incline reverse-grip dumbbell bench press	2 x 9–11
Arnold press	2 x 9–11
Cable face pull	3 x 9–11
Triceps dip*	2 x 9–11
Lying side hip raise*	2 x 20–25
Bicycle crunch	3 x 20–25
*To be performed as a superset	

Workout C (Legs and core)	
Exercise	Sets x Reps
Barbell squat	3 x 9–11
Dumbbell lunge	3 x 9–11
Inverse leg curl or lying leg curl	3 x 9–11
Machine seated calf raise	2 x 20–25
Machine standing calf raise*	2 x 20–25
Cable down-up twist*	2 x 9–11
Captain's chair leg and hip raise with dumbbell between feet	3 x 9–11
*To be performed as a superset	

Alternatives for cable/machine exercises

- Seated cable row — Bent-over dumbbell row, bent-over barbell row, or band row
- Wheel rollout — Ab walkout or inch worm

- Cable face pull — Band face pull or dumbbell face pull
- Triceps dip — Weighted bench dip
- Machine seated calf raise — Barbell seated calf raise
- Machine standing calf raise — Standing dumbbell one-leg calf raise or band standing calf raise
- Cable down-up twist — Band down-up twist or weighted Russian twist
- Captain's chair leg and hip raise with dumbbell between feet — Hanging leg and hip raise with dumbbell between feet or lying leg and hip raise with bands attached to ankles

Muscle 2

Description

The 8-week Muscle 2 program is designed to:

- train all of your major muscle groups
- build muscle in the 9–11 and 6–8 rep ranges
- strengthen your core and primal movement patterns
- introduce you to rep range alternation (undulating periodization)
- introduce you to the intensity technique of training to failure.

The program consists of two upper–lower splits, which means that there are four workouts (A, B, C, and D). Workouts A and C will train your upper body; workouts B and D will train your lower body.

In weeks 1, 3, 5, and 7, you will train in the 9–11 rep range; in weeks 2, 4, 6, and 8, you will train in the 6–8 rep range.

Please read the **Overview of men's training programs**, at the beginning of this chapter, to understand why you will be alternating rep ranges.

Suitability

- Lifters who have completed the Muscle program
- Anyone who has at least 6 months of consistent weight training experience

Instructions

- Complete the workouts (A, B, C, and D) in the order provided.
- The recommend workout schedule is ABXCDXX (where "X" represents a rest day). Try not to work out for four days in a row and have three days off.
- Complete the exercises in the order provided.
- Perform all of the sets for each exercise before moving on to the sets of the next exercise.
- Rest for 30 to 90 seconds between sets.

- Rest for 1 to 2 minutes between exercises.
- Try to master the proper form of each exercise, including proper breathing technique. Instructions for most exercises are available on my website, **weighttraining.guide**. Also, try to develop a mental connection with your muscles and the movement patterns.
- If you get bored of an exercise, see the **Overview of men's training programs** for alternatives.
- If training at home in the absence of cable machines and other specialized equipment, see below the exercise tables for exercise alternatives.
- Always use an amount of weight that will make hitting the rep range challenging.
- Whenever you have to increase the weight, add a maximum of 5 lb (2.5 kg) to upper-body exercises or 10 lb (5 kg) to lower-body exercises.
- In weeks 1, 3, 5, and 7, take the last set of every exercise to failure — that is, keep doing reps until you can't do another rep in good form. This is an intensity technique known as training to failure. Note that for some exercises, such as the barbell squat, you will not be able to safely train to failure unless you have a training partner or spotter ready, in which case do not train to failure.
- Don't forget to warm up before, and cool down after, each workout.
- Once you have completed the Muscle 2 program, you must take a deload week. Only then can you move on to the next program or redo the same program.

Workout A (Upper Body)		
Exercise	**Sets x Reps**	
	*Weeks 1, 3, 5, 7	Weeks 2, 4, 6, 8
Medium-grip lat pull-down	3 x 9–11	3 x 6–8
T-bar row	3 x 9–11	3 x 6–8
Dumbbell bench press	3 x 9–11	3 x 6–8
Seated dumbbell overhead press	2 x 9–11	2 x 6–8
Cable face pull	3 x 9–11	3 x 6–8
Triceps dip with a dumbbell between your feet	2 x 9–11	2 x 6–8
Dumbbell cross-body hammer curl	2 x 9–11	2 x 6–8
*If possible, take the last set of every exercise to failure		

Workout B (Lower Body)

Exercise	Sets x Reps	
	*Weeks 1, 3, 5, 7	Weeks 2, 4, 6, 8
Barbell sumo squat	3 x 9–11	3 x 6–8
Barbell one-leg hip thrust	2 x 9–11	2 x 6–8
Seated or lying leg curl	2 x 9–11	2 x 6–8
Standing dumbbell one-leg calf raise	3 x 20–25	3 x 15–20
Lying side hip raise	2 x 20–25	2 x 25–30
Bicycle crunch	3 x 20–25	3 x 25–30
One-leg front plank	2 x 60–90 s	2 x 60–90 s
*If possible, take the last set of every exercise to failure. s = seconds		

Workout C (Upper Body)

Exercise	Sets x Reps	
	*Weeks 1, 3, 5, 7	Weeks 2, 4, 6, 8
Cable twisting one-arm row	3 x 9–11	3 x 6–8
Barbell bench press	3 x 9–11	3 x 6–8
Incline reverse-grip dumbbell bench press	2 x 9–11	2 x 6–8
Dumbbell lateral raise	2 x 9–11	2 x 6–8
Dumbbell bent-over lateral raise	3 x 9–11	3 x 6–8
Decline EZ bar triceps extension	2 x 9–11	2 x 6–8
Incline dumbbell curl	3 x 9–11	3 x 6–8
*If possible, take the last set of every exercise to failure		

Workout D (Lower Body)

Exercise	Sets x Reps	
	*Weeks 1, 3, 5, 7	Weeks 2, 4, 6, 8
Barbell Romanian deadlift	3 x 9–11	3 x 6–8

Dumbbell Bulgarian split squat	2 x 9–11	2 x 6–8
Seated or lying leg curl	2 x 9–11	2 x 6–8
Machine seated calf raise	3 x 20–25	3 x 15–20
Cable wood chop	2 x 9–11	2 x 6–8
Captain's chair leg and hip raise with a dumbbell between feet	3 x 9–11	3 x 6–8
Wheel rollout	2 x 10–15	2 x 15–20
*If possible, take the last set of every exercise to failure		

Alternatives for cable/machine exercises

- Medium-grip lat pull-down — Medium-grip band lat pull-down or medium-grip pull-up
- T-bar row — Bent-over dumbbell row, bent-over barbell row, or band row
- Cable face pull — Band face pull or dumbbell face pull
- Triceps dip — Weighted bench dip
- Seated or lying leg curl — Inverse leg curl, one-leg stability ball leg curl, or band leg curl
- Cable twisting one-arm row — Band twisting one-arm row or dumbbell twisting row
- Machine seated calf raise — Barbell seated calf raise
- Cable wood chop — Band wood chop or weighted Russian twist
- Captain's chair leg and hip raise with dumbbell between feet — Hanging leg and hip raise with dumbbell between feet or lying leg and hip raise with bands attached to ankles
- Wheel rollout — Ab walkout or inch worm

Muscle and Strength

Description

The 12-week Muscle and Strength program is designed to:

- train all of your major muscle groups
- build muscle in the 9–11 and 6–8 rep ranges, and build strength in the 3–5 rep range
- strengthen your core and primal movement patterns
- introduce you to the intensity technique of dropset training.

The program consists of two pull–push splits, which means that there are four workouts (A, B, C, and D). Workouts A and C will train the pull muscles of your body; workouts B and D will train the push muscles of your body.

In weeks 1, 4, 7, and 10, you will train in the 9–11 rep range (muscle); in weeks 2, 5, 8, and 11, you will train in the 6–8 rep range (muscle); and in weeks 3, 6, 9, and 12, you will train in the 3–5 rep range (strength).

Please read the **Overview of men's training programs**, at the beginning of this chapter, before you start this program.

Suitability

- Lifters who have completed the Muscle 2 program
- Anyone who has at least 9 months of consistent weight training experience

Instructions

- Complete the workouts in the order provided.
- The recommend workout schedule is ABXCDXX (where "X" is a rest day). Try not to work out for four days in a row and have three days off.
- Complete the exercises in the order provided.
- Perform all of the sets for each exercise before moving on to the sets of the next exercise.
- During muscle weeks, rest for 30 to 90 seconds between sets and 1 to 2 minutes between exercises.
- During strength weeks, rest for 2 to 5 minutes between sets and 1 to 2 minutes between exercises.
- Try to master the proper form of each exercise, including proper breathing technique. Instructions for most exercises are available on my website, **weighttraining.guide**. Also, try to develop a mental connection with your muscles and the movement patterns.
- If you get bored of an exercise, see the **Overview of men's training programs** for alternatives.
- If training at home in the absence of cable machines and other specialized equipment, see below the exercise tables for exercise alternatives.
- Always use an amount of weight that will make hitting the rep range challenging.
- Whenever you have to increase the weight, add a maximum of 5 lb (2.5 kg) to upper-body exercises or 10 lb (5 kg) to lower-body exercises.
- In weeks 1, 4, 7, and 10, take the last set of every exercise to failure. Then, without resting, reduce the amount of weight on the bar and continue until failure again. This intensity technique is known as dropset training. Note that it is not safe to use it on some exercises, such as the barbell squat, unless you have a spotter. If you do not have a spotter, do not use the technique.
- Don't forget to warm up before, and cool down after, each workout.
- Once you have completed the Muscle and Strength program, you must take a deload week. Only then can you move on to the next program or redo the same program.

Workout A (Pull)			
	Sets x Reps		
Exercise	**Muscle weeks**		**Strength weeks**
	***Weeks 1, 4, 7, 10**	**Weeks 2, 5, 8, 11**	**Weeks 3, 6, 9, 12**
Barbell deadlift	3 x 9–11	3 x 6–8	3 x 3–5
Seated or lying leg curl	2 x 9–11	2 x 6–8	2 x 3–5
Seated cable row	3 x 9–11	3 x 6–8	3 x 3–5
Dumbbell bent-over lateral raise	3 x 9–11	3 x 6–8	3 x 3–5
EZ bar curl	3 x 9–11	3 x 6–8	3 x 3–5
Dumbbell Cuban rotation	2 x 15–20	2 x 15–20	2 x 10–15
Bicycle crunch	3 x 20–25	3 x 25–30	3 x 30–35
*If possible, perform a dropset for the last set of every exercise			

Workout B (Push)			
	Sets x Reps		
Exercise	**Muscle weeks**		**Strength weeks**
	***Weeks 1, 4, 7, 10**	**Weeks 2, 5, 8, 11**	**Weeks 3, 6, 9, 12**
Dumbbell lunge	3 x 9–11	3 x 6–8	3 x 3–5
Barbell hip thrust	2 x 9–11	2 x 6–8	2 x 3–5
Machine standing calf raise	3 x 20–25	3 x 15–20	3 x 10–15
Barbell bench press	3 x 9–11	3 x 6–8	3 x 3–5
Incline reverse-grip dumbbell bench press	2 x 9–11	2 x 6–8	2 x 3–5
Seated EZ bar overhead triceps extension	2 x 9–11	2 x 6–8	2 x 3–5
One-leg front plank	2 x 60–90 s	2 x 60–90 s	2 x 90–120 s
*If possible, perform a dropset for the last set of every exercise. s = seconds			

Workout C (Pull)			
	Sets x Reps		
Exercise	**Muscle weeks**		**Strength weeks**
	***Weeks 1, 4, 7, 10**	**Weeks 2, 5, 8, 11**	**Weeks 3, 6, 9, 12**
Pull-up with dumbbell between feet	3 x 9–11	3 x 6–8	3 x 3–5
Bent-over dumbbell row	2 x 9–11	2 x 6–8	2 x 3–5
Cable face pull	3 x 9–11	3 x 6–8	3 x 6–8
Dumbbell curl	3 x 9–11	3 x 6–8	3 x 3–5
Captain's chair leg and hip raise with dumbbell between feet	3 x 9–11	3 x 6–8	3 x 6–8
Wheel rollout	3 x 10–15	3 x 15–20	3 x 15–20
Twisting hyperextension holding a plate to chest	2 x 9–11	2 x 6–8	2 x 6–8
*If possible, perform a dropset for the last set of every exercise			

Workout D (Push)			
	Sets x Reps		
Exercise	**Muscle weeks**		**Strength weeks**
	***Weeks 1, 4, 7, 10**	**Weeks 2, 5, 8, 11**	**Weeks 3, 6, 9, 12**
Barbell squat	3 x 9–11	3 x 6–8	3 x 3–5
Machine seated calf raise	3 x 20–25	3 x 15–20	3 x 10–15
Hammer-grip dumbbell bench press	3 x 9–11	3 x 6–8	3 x 3–5
Low cable cross-over	2 x 9–11	2 x 6–8	2 x 3–5
Dumbbell one-arm overhead press	2 x 9–11	2 x 6–8	2 x 3–5
Triceps rope push-down	2 x 9–11	2 x 6–8	2 x 3–5
Lying side hip raise	2 x 20–25	2 x 25–30	2 x 30–35
*If possible, perform a dropset for the last set of every exercise			

Alternatives for cable/machine exercises

- Seated or lying leg curl — Inverse leg curl, one-leg stability ball leg curl, or band leg curl
- Seated cable row — Bent-over dumbbell row, bent-over barbell row, or band row
- Machine standing calf raise — Standing dumbbell one-leg calf raise or band standing calf raise
- Cable face pull — Band face pull or dumbbell face pull
- Captain's chair leg and hip raise with dumbbell between feet — Hanging leg and hip raise with dumbbell between feet or lying leg and hip raise with bands attached to ankles
- Wheel rollout — Ab walkout or inch worm
- Twisting hyperextension holding a plate to chest — Twisting hyperextension holding a plate to chest on flat bench
- Machine seated calf raise — Barbell seated calf raise
- Low cable cross-over — Incline dumbbell fly
- Triceps rope push-down — Barbell overhead triceps extension or band push-down

Muscle and Strength 2

Description

The 9-week Muscle and Strength 2 program is designed to:

- train all of your major muscle groups
- build muscle in the 9–11 and 6–8 rep ranges, and build strength in the 3–5 rep range
- strengthen your core and primal movement patterns
- introduce you to the intensity technique of rest–pause training.

The program consists of five workouts (A, B, C, D, and E). Workout A will train your back, biceps, and core; Workout B will train your chest, shoulders, triceps, and core; Workout C will train your legs and core; Workout D will train your upper body; and Workout E will train your lower body.

In weeks 1, 4, and 7, you will train in the 9–11 rep range (muscle); in weeks 2, 5, and 8, you will train in the 6–8 rep range (muscle); and in weeks 3, 6, and 9, you will train in the 3–5 rep range (strength).

Please read the **Overview of men's training programs**, at the beginning of this chapter, before you start this program.

Suitability

- Lifters who have completed the Muscle and Strength program
- Anyone who has at least 12 months of consistent weight training experience

Instructions

- Complete the workouts (A, B, C, D, and E) in the order provided.
- The recommend workout schedule is ABCXDEX (where "X" is a rest day). Try not to work out for five days in a row and have two days off.
- Complete the exercises in the order provided.
- During muscle weeks, rest for 30 to 90 seconds between sets and 1 to 2 minutes between exercises.
- During strength weeks, rest for 2 to 5 minutes between sets and 1 to 2 minutes between exercises.
- Try to master the proper form of each exercise, including proper breathing technique. Instructions for most exercises can be found on my website, **weighttraining.guide**. Also, try to develop a mental connection with your muscles and with the movement patterns.
- If you get bored of an exercise, see the **Overview of men's training programs** for alternatives.
- If training at home in the absence of cable machines and other specialized equipment, see below the exercise tables for exercise alternatives.
- Always use a weight that is heavy enough to make the reps challenging.
- Whenever you have to increase the weight, add a maximum of 5 lb (2.5 kg) to upper-body exercises or 10 lb (5 kg) to lower-body exercises.
- In weeks 1, 4, and 7, take the last set of every exercise to failure, put down the weights, wait for 15 to 20 seconds, pick the weights back up, and continue until you hit failure again. This intensity technique is known as rest–pause training. Note that it is not safe to use it on some exercises, such as the barbell squat, unless you have a spotter. If you do not have a spotter, please do not use the technique.
- Don't forget to warm up before, and cool down after, each workout.
- Once you have completed the Muscle and Strength 2 program, you must take a deload week. Only then can you move on to another program or redo the same program.

Workout A (Back, biceps, core)		
	Sets x Reps	
Exercise	Muscle weeks	Strength weeks
	*Weeks 1, 4, 7	Weeks 2, 5, 8	Weeks 3, 6, 9
Pull-up with dumbbell between feet	3 x 9–11	3 x 6–8	3 x 3–5
Cable twisting one-arm row	3 x 9–11	3 x 6–8	3 x 3–5
EZ bar curl	2 x 9–11	2 x 6–8	2 x 3–5
EZ bar reverse curl	2 x 9–11	2 x 6–8	2 x 3–5
Dumbbell lying external shoulder rotation	2 x 15–20	2 x 15–20	2 x 10–15

Bicycle crunch	3 x 20–25	3 x 25–30	3 x 30–35
Lying side hip raise	2 x 20–25	2 x 25–30	2 x 30–35

*If possible, perform a rest pause for the last set of every exercise

Workout B (Chest, shoulders, triceps, core)			
	Sets x Reps		
Exercise	Muscle weeks		Strength weeks
	*Weeks 1, 4, 7	Weeks 2, 5, 8	Weeks 3, 6, 9
Barbell bench press	3 x 9–11	3 x 6–8	3 x 3–5
Incline reverse-grip dumbbell bench press	3 x 9–11	3 x 6–8	3 x 3–5
Barbell overhead press	3 x 9–11	3 x 6–8	3 x 3–5
Wide-grip barbell upright row	2 x 9–11	2 x 6–8	2 x 3–5
Cable face pull	3 x 9–11	3 x 6–8	3 x 6–8
Triceps dip with dumbbell between feet	2 x 9–11	2 x 6–8	2 x 3–5
One-leg front plank	2 x 60–90 s	2 x 60–90 s	2 x 90–120 s

*If possible, perform a rest pause for the last set of every exercise. s = seconds

Workout C (Legs and core)			
	Sets x Reps		
Exercise	Muscle weeks		Strength weeks
	*Weeks 1, 4, 7	Weeks 2, 5, 8	Weeks 3, 6, 9
Barbell squat	3 x 9–11	3 x 6–8	3 x 3–5
Dumbbell side lunge	2 x 9–11	2 x 6–8	2 x 3–5
Seated or lying leg curl	3 x 9–11	3 x 6–8	3 x 3–5
Machine standing calf raise	3 x 20–25	3 x 15–20	3 x 10–15
Machine seated calf raise	2 x 20–25	2 x 15–20	2 x 10–15

142

Hanging leg and hip raise holding a dumbbell between feet	3 x 9–11	3 x 6–8	3 x 6–8
Cable twist	2 x 9–11	2 x 6–8	2 x 6–8

*If possible, perform a rest pause for the last set of every exercise

Workout D (Upper body)			
	Sets x Reps		
Exercise	**Muscle weeks**		**Strength weeks**
	*Weeks 1, 4, 7	Weeks 2, 5, 8	Weeks 3, 6, 9
Weighted inverted row	3 x 9–11	3 x 6–8	3 x 3–5
One-arm lat pull-down	2 x 9–11	2 x 6–8	2 x 3–5
Weighted push-up or hammer-grip dumbbell bench press	3 x 9–11	3 x 6–8	3 x 3–5
Low cable cross-over	2 x 9–11	2 x 6–8	2 x 3–5
Dumbbell bent-over lateral raise	3 x 9–11	3 x 6–8	3 x 3–5
Cable triceps kickback	3 x 9–11	3 x 6–8	3 x 3–5
Incline dumbbell curl	2 x 9–11	2 x 6–8	2 x 3–5

*If possible, perform a rest pause for the last set of every exercise

Workout E (Lower body)			
	Sets x Reps		
Exercise	**Muscle weeks**		**Strength weeks**
	*Weeks 1, 4, 7	Weeks 2, 5, 8	Weeks 3, 6, 9
Barbell deadlift	3 x 9–11	3 x 6–8	3 x 3–5
Dumbbell Bulgarian split squat	2 x 9–11	2 x 6–8	2 x 3–5
Barbell hip thrust	2 x 9–11	2 x 6–8	2 x 3–5
Seated or lying leg curl	2 x 9–11	2 x 6–8	2 x 3–5
Machine standing calf raise	3 x 20–25	3 x 15–20	3 x 10–15

Wheel rollout	3 x 10–15	3 x 15–20	3 x 15–20
Horizontal Pallof press	2 x 9–11	2 x 6–8	2 x 6–8
*If possible, perform a rest pause for the last set of every exercise			

Alternatives for cable/machine exercises

- Cable twisting one-arm row — Band twisting one-arm row or dumbbell twisting row
- Cable face pull — Band face pull or dumbbell face pull
- Triceps dip — Weighted bench dip
- Seated or lying leg curl — Inverse leg curl, one-leg stability ball leg curl, or band leg curl
- Machine standing calf raise — Standing dumbbell one-leg calf raise or band standing calf raise
- Machine seated calf raise — Barbell seated calf raise
- Cable twist — Weighted Russian twist or band twist
- Weighted inverted row — Bent-over barbell row or seated band row
- One-arm lat pull-down — Pull-up or one-arm band lat pull-down
- Low cable cross-over — Incline dumbbell fly
- Cable triceps kickback — Band triceps kickback or skull crusher
- Wheel rollout — Ab walkout or inch worm
- Horizontal Pallof press — Band horizontal Pallof press or weighted lying oblique twist

Muscle and Strength 3

Description

The 12-week Muscle and Strength 3 program is designed to:

- train all of your major muscle groups
- build muscle in the 9–11 and 6–8 rep ranges, and build strength in the 3–5 rep range
- strengthen your core and primal movement patterns
- increase training intensity and volume (the number of exercises and sets that you perform) while reducing the amount of time that you spend in the gym.

The program consists of four workouts (A, B, C, and D). Workouts A and C will train your upper body and core; workouts B and D will train your lower body and core.

The exercises in all of the workouts have been arranged into supersets, which makes the workouts both shorter and more intense than the workouts of preceding programs.

In weeks 1, 4, 7, and 10, you will train in the 9–11 rep range (muscle); in weeks 2, 5, 8, and 11, you will train in the 6–8 rep range (muscle); and in weeks 3, 6, 9, and 12, you will train in the 3–5 rep range (strength).

Please read the **Overview of men's training programs**, at the beginning of this chapter, before you start this program.

Suitability

- Individuals who have completed the Muscle and Strength 2 program
- Anyone who has at least 12 months of consistent weight training experience

Instructions

- Complete the workouts (A, B, C, and D) in the order presented.
- The recommend workout schedule is ABXCDXX (where "X" is a rest day). Try not to work out for four days in a row and rest for three days.
- The exercises are arranged into pairs as supersets. After you complete one set of the first exercise, perform a set of the second exercise without resting.
- During muscle weeks, rest for 1 to 2 minutes before repeating the superset and before moving on to the next superset.
- During strength weeks, rest for 2 to 5 minutes before repeating the superset and before moving on to the next superset.
- Always use a weight that is heavy enough to make the reps challenging.
- Whenever you have to increase the weight, add a maximum of 5 lb (2.5 kg) to upper-body exercises or 10 lb (5 kg) to lower-body exercises.
- Try to master the proper form of each exercise, including proper breathing technique. Instructions for most exercises can be found on my website, **weighttraining.guide**. Also, try to develop a mental connection with your muscles and with the movement patterns.
- If you get bored of an exercise, see the **Overview of men's training programs** for alternatives.
- If training at home in the absence of cable machines and other specialized equipment, see below the exercise tables for exercise alternatives.
- Don't forget to warm up before, and cool down after, each workout.
- Once you have completed Muscle and Strength 3, you must take a deload week. Only then can you repeat the program or one of the other programs.

Workout A (Upper body and core)			
	Sets x Reps		
Exercise	**Muscle weeks**		**Strength weeks**
	Weeks 1, 4, 7, 10	Weeks 2, 5, 8, 11	Weeks 3, 6, 9, 12
Bent-over barbell row	2 x 9–11	2 x 6–8	2 x 3–5
Barbell bench press	2 x 9–11	2 x 6–8	2 x 3–5

Exercise			
Weighted inverted row, underhand grip	2 x 9–11	2 x 6–8	2 x 3–5
Weighted push-up or Dumbbell bench press	2 x 9–11	2 x 6–8	2 x 3–5
Medium-grip lat pull-down	3 x 9–11	3 x 6–8	3 x 3–5
Dumbbell one-arm overhead press	3 x 9–11	3 x 6–8	3 x 3–5
Dumbbell curl	2 x 9–11	2 x 6–8	2 x 3–5
Overhead barbell triceps extension	2 x 9–11	2 x 6–8	2 x 3–5
One-leg front plank	2 x 60–90 s	2 x 60–90 s	2 x 90–120 s

s = seconds

Workout B (Lower body and core)

Exercise	Sets x Reps		
	Muscle weeks		Strength weeks
	Weeks 1, 4, 7, 10	Weeks 2, 5, 8, 11	Weeks 3, 6, 9, 12
Barbell squat	3 x 9–11	3 x 6–8	3 x 3–5
Dumbbell Romanian deadlift	3 x 9–11	3 x 6–8	3 x 3–5
Dumbbell lunge	2 x 9–11	2 x 6–8	2 x 3–5
Bicycle crunch	2 x 20–25	2 x 25–30	2 x 30–35
Barbell hip thrust	2 x 9–11	2 x 6–8	2 x 3–5
Captain's chair leg and hip raise with dumbbell between feet	2 x 9–11	2 x 6–8	2 x 6–8
Machine standing calf raise	3 x 20–25	3 x 15–20	3 x 10–15
Wheel rollout	3 x 10–15	3 x 15–20	3 x 15–20

Workout C (Upper body)

Exercise	Sets x Reps		
	Muscle weeks		Strength weeks
	Weeks 1, 4, 7, 10	Weeks 2, 5, 8, 11	Weeks 3, 6, 9, 12
Seated cable row	3 x 9–11	3 x 6–8	3 x 3–5
Triceps dip with dumbbell between feet	3 x 9–11	3 x 6–8	3 x 3–5
One-arm standing twisting cable row	2 x 9–11	2 x 6–8	2 x 3–5

One-arm standing twisting cable chest press	2 x 9–11	2 x 6–8	2 x 3–5
Dumbbell bent-over lateral raise	2 x 9–11	2 x 6–8	2 x 3–5
Dumbbell fly	2 x 9–11	2 x 6–8	2 x 3–5
Barbell reverse curl	2 x 9–11	2 x 6–8	2 x 3–5
Triceps rope push-down	2 x 9–11	2 x 6–8	2 x 3–5
Cable face pull	3 x 9–11	3 x 6–8	3 x 6–8

Workout D (Lower body and core)			
	Sets x Reps		
Exercise	**Muscle weeks**		**Strength weeks**
	Weeks 1, 4, 7, 10	**Weeks 2, 5, 8, 11**	**Weeks 3, 6, 9, 12**
Barbell deadlift	3 x 9–11	3 x 6–8	3 x 3–5
Decline twisting sit-up	3 x 20–25	3 x 25–30	3 x 30–35
Dumbbell Bulgarian split squat	2 x 9–11	2 x 6–8	2 x 3–5
Single straight-leg dumbbell deadlift	2 x 9–11	2 x 6–8	2 x 3–5
Leg extension	2 x 9–11	2 x 6–8	2 x 6–8
Seated or lying leg curl	2 x 9–11	2 x 6–8	2 x 3–5
Machine seated calf raise	3 x 20–25	3 x 15–20	3 x 10–15
Hanging straight leg and hip raise	3 x 9–11	3 x 12–14	3 x 15–18

Alternatives for cable/machine exercises

- Weighted inverted row — Bent-over barbell row or seated band row
- Medium-grip lat pull-down — Medium-grip band lat pull-down or medium-grip pull-up
- Captain's chair leg and hip raise with dumbbell between feet — Hanging leg and hip raise with dumbbell between feet or lying leg and hip raise with bands attached to ankles
- Machine standing calf raise — Standing dumbbell one-leg calf raise or band standing calf raise
- Wheel rollout — Ab walkout or inch worm
- Seated cable row — Bent-over dumbbell row, bent-over barbell row, or band row
- Triceps dip — Weighted bench dip
- One-arm standing twisting cable row — One-arm standing twisting band row or dumbbell twisting row
- One-arm standing twisting chest press — One-arm standing twisting chest press with band or one-arm dumbbell bench press
- Triceps rope push-down — Skull crusher or triceps band push-down

- Cable face pull — Band face pull or dumbbell face pull
- Leg extension — Sissy squat
- Seated or lying leg curl — Inverse leg curl, one-leg stability ball leg curl, or band leg curl
- Machine seated calf raise — Barbell seated calf raise

Men's Plateau Buster

Description

The 9-week Men's Plateau Buster is designed to:

- train all of your major muscle groups
- build muscle in the 9–11 and 6–8 rep ranges, and build strength in the 3–5 rep range
- strengthen your core and primal movement patterns
- introduce you to the pre-exhaustion intensity training protocol
- help you to break out of plateaus and keep making progress.

The program consists of three workouts (A, B, and C). Workout A will train your back, biceps, and core; Workout B will train your chest, shoulders, and triceps; and Workout C will train your legs and core.

In weeks 1, 4, and 7, you will train in the 9–11 rep range (muscle); in weeks 2, 5, and 8, you will train in the 6–8 rep range (muscle); and in weeks 3, 6, and 9, you will train in the 3–5 rep range (strength).

The exercises in each workout have been arranged in accordance with the pre-exhaustion protocol, which will ensure that your prime mover muscles are partially exhausted by isolation exercises before you move on to the major compound exercises. The pre-exhaustion is intended to boost muscular overload and amplify the stimulus for development, thus increasing the program's chances of helping you to "bust" through plateaus and keep making progress. You can also use the program as an additional and advanced Muscle and Strength mesocycle ("Muscle and Strength 4").

Please read the **Overview of men's training programs**, at the beginning of this chapter, before you start this program.

Suitability

- Individuals who have completed the Muscle and Strength 3 program
- Anyone who has at least 12 months of consistent weight training experience

Instructions

- Complete the workouts (A, B, and C) in the order presented.

- The recommend workout schedules are ABCX (i.e. three days on, one day off) or ABCXABX (i.e. three days on, one day off, two days on, one day off, and then continue the sequence from where you left off).
- Perform the exercises in the order presented.
- During muscle weeks, rest for 30 to 90 seconds between sets and 1 to 2 minutes between exercises.
- During strength weeks, rest for 2 to 5 minutes between sets and 1 to 2 minutes between exercises.
- Always use a weight that is heavy enough to make the reps challenging.
- Whenever you have to increase the weight, add a maximum of 5 lb (2.5 kg) to upper-body exercises or 10 lb (5 kg) to lower-body exercises.
- Try to master the proper form of each exercise, including proper breathing technique. Instructions for most exercises are available on my website, **weighttraining.guide**. Also, try to develop a mental connection with your muscles and with the movement patterns.
- If you get bored of an exercise, see the **Overview of men's training programs** for alternatives.
- If training at home in the absence of cable machines and other specialized equipment, see below the exercise tables for exercise alternatives.
- Don't forget to warm up before, and cool down after, each workout.
- Once you have completed the Men's Plateau Buster, you must take a deload week. Only then can you repeat the program or one of the other programs.

Workout A (Back, biceps, core)			
	Sets x Reps		
Exercise	**Muscle weeks**		**Strength weeks**
	Weeks 1, 4, 7	**Weeks 2, 5, 8**	**Weeks 3, 6, 9**
Cable straight-arm pull-down	2 x 9–11	2 x 6–8	2 x 3–5
Pull-up with dumbbell between feet	2 x 9–11	2 x 6–8	2 x 3–5
One-arm twisting cable row	2 x 9–11	2 x 6–8	2 x 3–5
Bent-over barbell row using underhand grip	3 x 9–11	3 x 6–8	3 x 3–5
Dumbbell concentration curl	2 x 9–11	2 x 6–8	2 x 3–5
EZ bar curl	2 x 9–11	2 x 6–8	2 x 3–5
Wheel rollout	3 x 10–15	3 x 15–20	3 x 15–20
Bicycle crunch	3 x 20–25	3 x 25–30	3 x 30–35
Dumbbell side bend	2 x 20–25	2 x 15–20	2 x 10–15

Workout B (Chest, shoulders, triceps)			
	Sets x Reps		
Exercise	Muscle weeks		Strength weeks
	Weeks 1, 4, 7	Weeks 2, 5, 8	Weeks 3, 6, 9
Dumbbell fly	2 x 9–11	2 x 6–8	2 x 3–5
Incline reverse-grip dumbbell bench press	2 x 9–11	2 x 6–8	2 x 3–5
Barbell bench press	3 x 9–11	3 x 6–8	3 x 3–5
Alternating dumbbell front raise	2 x 9–11	2 x 6–8	2 x 3–5
Barbell overhead press	2 x 9–11	2 x 6–8	2 x 3–5
Dumbbell bent-over lateral raise	2 x 9–11	2 x 6–8	2 x 3–5
Cable face pull	3 x 9–11	3 x 6–8	3 x 6–8
Overhead barbell triceps extension	2 x 9–11	2 x 6–8	2 x 3–5
Triceps dip with dumbbell between feet	2 x 9–11	2 x 6–8	2 x 3–5

Workout C (Legs and core)			
	Sets x Reps		
Exercise	Muscle weeks		Strength weeks
	Weeks 1, 4, 7	Weeks 2, 5, 8	Weeks 3, 6, 9
Leg extension	2 x 9–11	2 x 6–8	2 x 6–8
Barbell hip thrust	2 x 9–11	2 x 6–8	2 x 3–5
Barbell squat	3 x 9–11	3 x 6–8	3 x 3–5
Seated or lying leg curl	2 x 9–11	2 x 6–8	2 x 3–5
Twisting hyperextension holding plate against chest	2 x 9–11	2 x 6–8	2 x 6–8
Barbell Romanian deadlift	2 x 9–11	2 x 6–8	2 x 3–5
Machine seated calf raise	2 x 20–25	2 x 15–20	2 x 10–15
Machine standing calf raise	3 x 20–25	3 x 15–20	3 x 10–15
Captain's chair leg and hip raise with dumbbell between feet	3 x 9–11	3 x 6–8	3 x 6–8

Alternatives for cable/machine exercises

- Cable straight-arm pull-down — Band straight-arm pull-down or dumbbell pull-over
- One-arm twisting cable row — One-arm twisting band row or dumbbell twisting row
- Wheel rollout — Ab walkout or inch worm
- Cable face pull — Band face pull or dumbbell face pull
- Triceps dip — Weighted bench dip
- Leg extension — Sissy squat
- Seated or lying leg curl — Inverse leg curl, one-leg stability ball leg curl, or band leg curl
- Twisting hyperextension holding plate against chest — Twisting hyperextension on flat bench holding plate against chest
- Machine seated calf raise — Barbell seated calf raise
- Machine standing calf raise — Standing dumbbell one-leg calf raise or band standing calf raise
- Captain's chair leg and hip raise with dumbbell between feet — Hanging leg and hip raise with dumbbell between feet or lying leg and hip raise with bands strapped to ankles

Minimalistic Program for Busy Men

Description

The 12-week Minimalistic Program for Busy Men is designed to:

- train all of your major muscle groups
- build muscle in the 9–11 and 6–8 rep ranges
- strengthen your core and primal movement patterns
- introduce you to the intensity technique of superset training
- minimize the time it takes to get an effective full-body workout.

The program consists of two workouts (A and B). Workout A will train your upper body and core; Workout B will train your lower body and core.

The exercises in all of the workouts have been arranged into supersets, which makes the workouts short and intense.

In weeks 1, 3, 5, 7, 9, and 11, you will train in the 9–11 rep range; in weeks 2, 4, 6, 8, 10, and 12, you will train in the 6–8 rep range.

Please read the **Overview of men's training programs**, at the beginning of this chapter, before you start this program.

Suitability

- Individuals who have completed at least microcycles 1–3 of the Men's Beginner program

- Anyone who has at least 3 months of consistent weight training experience

Instructions

- Complete each workout (A and B) twice per week, in the order presented.
- The recommend workout schedule is ABXABXX (where "X" is a rest day). Try not to train for four days in a row and rest for three days (i.e. ABABXXX).
- The exercises are arranged into pairs as supersets. After you complete one set of the first exercise, perform a set of the second exercise without resting.
- Rest for 1 to 2 minutes before repeating the superset and before moving on to the next superset.
- Always use a weight that is heavy enough to make the reps challenging.
- Whenever you have to increase the weight, add a maximum of 5 lb (2.5 kg) to upper-body exercises or 10 lb (5 kg) to lower-body exercises.
- Try to master the proper form of each exercise, including proper breathing technique. Instructions for most exercises are available on my website, **weighttraining.guide**. Also, try to develop a mental connection with your muscles and with the movement patterns.
- If you get bored of an exercise, see the **Overview of men's training programs** for alternatives.
- If training at home in the absence of cable machines and other specialized equipment, see below the exercise tables for exercise alternatives.
- Don't forget to warm up before, and cool down after, each workout.
- Once you have completed the Minimalistic Program for Busy Men, you must take a deload week (a week during which you either rest or train lightly). Only then can you repeat the program or start the Muscle and Strength programs from a suitable level.

Workout A (Upper body and core)		
Exercise	**Sets x Reps**	
	Weeks 1, 3, 5, 7, 9, 11	**Weeks 2, 4, 6, 8, 10, 12**
Bent-over two-arm dumbbell row	2 x 9–11	2 x 6–8
Dumbbell bench press	2 x 9–11	2 x 6–8
Medium-grip lat pull-down	2 x 9–11	2 x 6–8
Seated dumbbell overhead press	2 x 9–11	2 x 6–8
Cable face pull	2 x 9–11	2 x 6–8
Triceps dip with dumbbell between feet	2 x 9–11	2 x 6–8
Dumbbell curl	2 x 9–11	2 x 6–8
Wheel rollout	2 x 10–15	2 x 15–20

152

Workout B (Lower body and core)		
Exercise	**Sets x Reps**	
	Weeks 1, 3, 5, 7, 9, 11	**Weeks 2, 4, 6, 8, 10, 12**
Barbell squat	2 x 9–11	2 x 6–8
Dumbbell Romanian deadlift	2 x 9–11	2 x 6–8
Dumbbell lunge	2 x 9–11	2 x 6–8
Seated or lying leg curl	2 x 9–11	2 x 6–8
Captain's chair leg and hip raise	2 x 10–15	2 x 15–20
Machine standing calf raise	2 x 15–20	2 x 10–15
Bicycle crunch	2 x 25–30	2 x 30–35

Alternatives for cable/machine exercises

- Medium-grip lat pull-down — Medium-grip band lat pull-down or medium-grip pull-up
- Cable face pull — Band face pull or dumbbell face pull
- Triceps dip — Weighted bench dip
- Wheel rollout — Ab walkout or inch worm
- Seated or lying leg curl — Inverse leg curl, one-leg stability ball leg curl, or band leg curl
- Captain's chair leg and hip raise — Lying or hanging leg and hip raise
- Machine standing calf raise — Standing dumbbell one-leg calf raise or band standing calf raise

Chapter 8: Women's weight training programs

Overview of women's training programs

Programs for women

As summarized in Table 8.1, there are three weight training programs for women.

Program	Mesocycle	Duration (weeks)	Workouts Per Week	Workout duration (mins)	Repeatable?
Maximum Curves and Functional Strength (MCFS)	Women's Beginner	12	3-5	30–40	No
	MCFS 1	8	5	45–50	Yes
	MCFS 2	10	4	45–50	Yes
	MCFS 3	10	4	45–50	Yes
	MCFS 4	8	5	45–50	Yes
	MCFS 5	12	4	40–45	Yes
Women's Plateau Buster	N/A	8	5	55–60	Yes
Minimalistic Program for Busy Women	N/A	12	4	25–30	Yes

Table 8.1. Summary of the three weight training programs for women, including each program's duration, number of workouts per week, approximate workout duration, and whether or not the program can be repeated. The workout duration does not include the warmup and cooldown.

The first program, **Maximum Curves and Functional Strength (MCFS)**, actually consists of six smaller programs (mesocycles). As its name implies, MCFS is intended for women who want to develop maximum curves and a functionally strong body.

The **Women's Plateau Buster** is a stand-alone program that you can use if you ever experience a plateau (a plateau is when you stop making progress due to your body becoming adapted to the training stimulus). Since the program is designed to produce the same results as MCFS, you can also include it as part of MCFS and use it after MCFS 5.

The **Minimalistic Program for Busy Women** is another stand-alone program. It is designed to provide a quick and effective full-body workout for women who have very little time to spare for the gym.

You can complete the training programs at any gym or at home using the alternative exercises that I have provided for each program and the following equipment:

- Adjustable bench
- Dumbbells
- Pull-up bar
- Barbell
- Power rack for safety
- Clip resistance bands (optional but important in the absence of a cable machine and leg-curling machine)
- Ankle straps (optional but important for leg curls in the absence of a leg-curling machine, as well as inner- and outer-thigh exercises)
- Ab wheel (optional)
- Stability ball (optional)
- Loop band (optional)
- Dip bars (optional)

All of the programs and the way they were designed will be explored in detail below.

General instructions

If a beginner, you should start from the beginner program, after which you can move on to either the MCFS programs or the minimalistic program, depending on your preferences.

If experienced, you can start from any program that you choose as long as you meet the suitability criteria (see tables 8.2 and 8.3).

Maximum Curves and Functional Strength (MCFS)

MCFS is a comprehensive long-term weight training program that was meticulously designed to:

- develop and maintain major "curves"
- strengthen your body's primal movement patterns, thus improving your functional strength, balance, coordination, athleticism, and performance
- strengthen your core, which is important for stability, body-wide strength, power generation, and power transfer
- encourage the right strength balances between your opposing muscle groups, which is important for proper posture and movement, and to prevent imbalance-related injuries

The program achieves this by incorporating, or adhering to, a combination of:

- major compound (multi-joint) exercises
- functional exercises
- intensity training techniques

- undulating periodization
- recommended muscle strength balance ratios.

In programming terminology, MCFS is a **macrocycle** ("big cycle"). The six individual programs that make up MCFS (from the Women's Beginner program to MCFS 5) are known as **mesocycles** ("middle cycles"). Although not expressed in Table 8.1, most of the mesocycles are themselves divided into **microcycles** ("small cycles"). The mesocycles and microcycles incorporate variations in training, which will be explained in the mesocycle overview.

MCFS lasts for a minimum of one year and 13 weeks if you move from mesocycle to mesocycle and take a deload week after each one. A deload week is a week during which you either rest or train lightly. However, apart from the Women's Beginner mesocycle, you do not have to move from one mesocycle straight on to the next one. I balanced the exercises in each mesocycle as best as I could so that you can keep repeating each mesocycle over and over without much of a risk of developing muscular imbalances. As such, you can repeat each mesocycle as many times as you want to before moving on to the next one. This will ensure that you get the most out of each mesocycle and the macrocycle as a whole.

In fact, you don't have to move on at all. If you enjoy a particular mesocycle, you can stick to it. Provided you keep increasing the amount of weight that you lift, as requested in the instructions of each mesocycle, you should see continual progress for a significant amount of time. Just make sure that you take a deload week before repeating a mesocycle or moving on to the next mesocycle.

Note that the deload weeks are important. Please do not ignore them. They will help you to fully recover and therefore keep making progress. They will also increase your likelihood of not giving up.

Mesocycle overview

Women's Beginner

Before I provide an overview of each mesocycle (Table 8.2), I remind you that training in different rep ranges leads to the development of different muscle properties. More specifically, using a weight with which you can perform 13–20 reps in good form is optimal for developing muscular endurance; using a weight with which you can only perform 6–12 reps in good form (i.e. a heavy weight) is optimal for developing muscular size; and using a weight with which you can only perform 2–6 reps in good form (i.e. a very heavy weight) is optimal for developing muscular strength.

Focusing mostly on the 13+ rep range, the 12-week Women's Beginner mesocycle is designed to build a strong foundation of muscular endurance upon which muscular size can be built in the more advanced mesocycles. It is intended for beginners, individuals who have less than three months of consistent weight training experience, and experienced gym-goers who haven't trained for over three months.

Mesocycle	Rep ranges	Intensity technique	Experience required
Women's Beginner	13+	None	None
MCFS 1	9–11	Supersets	3 months
MCFS 2	9–11, 6–8	Training to failure	6 months
MCFS 3	9–11, 6–8	Dropsets	6 months
MCFS 4	9–11, 6–8	Rest–pause sets	9 months
MCFS 5	9–11, 6–8	Supersets	12 months

Table 8.2. The rep ranges and intensity techniques of each MCFS mesocycle, along with the level of experience required to start from each mesocycle.

MCFS 1

The 8-week MCFS 1 mesocycle starts to build muscle in the 9–11 rep range. It also incorporates an intensity technique known as **superset training**. You can start from this mesocycle without having to go through the Women's Beginner mesocycle only if you have at least three months of consistent weight training experience.

MCFS 2

The 10-week MCFS 2 mesocycle is composed of microcycles that alternate between the 9–11 and 6–8 rep ranges (you will learn below why rep ranges are alternated). This mesocycle includes an intensity technique known as **training to failure**. You can start from this mesocycle only if you have at least six months of consistent training experience.

MCFS 3

Like MCFS 2, the 10-week MCFS 3 mesocycle consists of microcycles that alternate between the 9–11 and 6–8 rep ranges. The mesocycle includes an intensity technique called **dropset training**. As with MCFS 2, you can start from this mesocycle only if you have at least six months of consistent weight training experience.

MCFS 4

As with MCFS 2 and MCFS 3, the 8-week MCFS 4 mesocycle consists of microcycles that alternate between the 9–11 and 6–8 rep ranges. It includes an intensity technique known as **rest–pause training**. You can start from this mesocycle only if you have at least nine months of consistent training experience.

MCFS 5

Although the 12-week MCFS 5 mesocycle also comprises microcycles that alternate between the 9–11 and 6–8 rep ranges, it is different from the other mesocycles in that all of the exercises are arranged into supersets. As such, the workouts are more intense and quicker to complete. You can start from this mesocycle only if you have at least 12 months of consistent weight training experience.

Why alternate between rep ranges?

The process of alternating rep ranges in microcycles is known as **undulating periodization**. Since training in different rep ranges leads to the development of different muscle properties (endurance, size, or strength), undulating periodization will help you to simultaneously develop and maintain different muscle properties.

In this instance, you will mostly be alternating between the 9–11 and 6–8 rep ranges, which are both primarily for building muscle. However, the 9–11 rep range will help you to develop muscular size and maintain a bit of endurance, while the 6–8 rep range will help you to develop muscular size and more strength. The extra strength will assist you in lifting heavier weights, which will help your muscles to grow, which will in turn help you to lift even heavier weights — thus promoting a cycle of growth.

I could have had you also alternate the 13+ rep range for maintaining the endurance that you develop in the Women's Beginner mesocycle, or I could have had you also alternate a 3–5 rep range for developing maximum strength. However, the endurance rep range would have significantly increased the time that it takes for you to build shape and curves (muscle), and the maximum strength rep range just doesn't appeal to most women.

Overview of the other training programs for women

Women's Plateau Buster

The 8-week Women's Plateau Buster is your weapon for breaking out of plateaus, should they ever occur. You can also use it as if it's the seventh MCFS mesocycle, and repeat it as many times as you want to.

As with the MCFS mesocycles, the Women's Plateau Buster consists of microcycles that alternate between the 9–11 and 6–8 rep ranges (Table 8.3). The difference is that most of the exercises are arranged in accordance with an advanced intensity protocol known as **pre-exhaustion training**, which will ensure that you partially exhaust prime mover muscles using isolation exercises before you move on to the main compound exercises. Pre-exhaustion of prime movers makes them work much harder during the compound exercises, thus amplifying the stimulus for development and increasing your chances of kick-starting stunted progress.

If you're new to weight training and follow MCFS, you will almost certainly not need this program as a plateau buster for at least a couple of years. However, if you ever do need it, it should ensure that you never stop making progress.

Program	Rep ranges	Intensity technique	Experience required
Women's Plateau Buster	9–11, 6–8	Pre-exhaustion	12 months
Minimalistic Program for Busy Women	9–11, 6–8	Supersets	Completion of microcycles 1–3 of the Women's Beginner mesocycle

Table 8.3. The rep ranges and intensity techniques of the women's plateau buster and minimalistic programs, along with the level of experience required to start from each program.

Minimalistic Program for Busy Women

The 12-week Minimalistic Program for Busy Women is for you if you don't have much time for workouts. Alternating between the 9–11 and 6–8 rep ranges, the workouts include the bare minimum of exercises and sets necessary to get an effective full-body workout and try to promote continual development. What's more, the exercises are arranged into supersets, which means that you can fly through them very rapidly.

Apart from a few basic adjustments to emphasize glute development, the Minimalistic Program for Busy Women is similar to the Minimalistic Program for Busy Men. As such, although it should take you quite far in terms of developing shape, it will not give you the kind of curves that you could get with MCFS.

You can repeat the Minimalistic Program for Busy Women as many times as you want to. If a beginner, ideally, before you start the program, you should have completed at least microcycles 1 through 3 of the Women's Beginner mesocycle. As with the minimalistic workouts, the workouts of microcycles 1 through 3 of the Women's Beginner mesocycle are short, and they will help you to develop a small foundation of muscular endurance upon which the Minimalistic Program for Busy Women can build.

How do the women's programs differ from the men's ones?

Men and women usually train for different goals. Men usually want maximum muscle and strength, whereas women usually want maximum shape and "tone". The training programs have been adapted to meet these different needs by incorporating different exercises and rep ranges.

It's important to realize that maximum muscle (one of men's goals) and maximum shape and tone (women's goals) are actually achieved by doing the same two things:

1. Losing body fat
2. Adding muscle to specific areas of the body

Therefore, the men's and women's training programs follow the same primary strength and conditioning principles.

Ladies, this means that you have to train (and eat) for muscle growth, just like the men have to. In other words, in order to develop the shape and tone that you want, you have to lose the light dumbbells and hit heavier weights!

Will heavy lifting make me look bulky, like a man?

No, because women generally possess ten times less testosterone than men do, so you should never expect to grow as muscular as a man unless you take testosterone artificially. Also, women add muscle at a slower rate than men do, which means that you have more than enough time to notice that you are getting too muscular and adjust your training.

Important!

Ladies, please do not be scared of heavy lifting. *This fear will prevent you from getting the results that you want!* If you want shape and tone, you have to build muscle in all of the right areas of your body, and the only way to do that is to lift heavier weights.

How the programs were designed

Exercise selection

The goals of all of the weight training programs for women are to develop and maintain curves and functional strength, strengthen the body's primal movement patterns, strengthen the core, and encourage the right strength balances between opposing muscle groups. Most of the exercises used in the programs were selected to meet those objectives. I explain how below. However, some exercises were included for other purposes, such as to prepare you in one mesocycle for more advanced exercises in the following mesocycle, or simply to add variation to the workouts to keep you engaged.

Balancing the exercises

When designing long-term training programs that will be repeated over and over, you must select exercises that promote appropriate strength balances between opposing muscle groups. The reason is that if opposing muscle groups develop significantly different strengths, the risk of sustaining injuries and developing problems related to muscle tightness, joint instability, and posture will be increased.

In order to reduce your likelihood of developing imbalances using the programs in this book, I designed them in accordance with the muscle strength balance ratios recommended by the International Fitness Professionals Association (IFPA; Table 8.4).

Muscle group	Muscle balance ratio
Hip flexors and extensors	1:1
Knee flexors and extensors	2:3

Shoulder flexors and extensors	2:3
Shoulder internal and external rotators	3:2
Elbow flexors and extensors	1:1
Trunk flexors and extensors	1:1
Ankle plantar flexors and dorsiflexors	3:1

Table 8.4. Muscle strength balance ratios recommended by the IFPA.

The strategy that I used was to:

- make note of the target and synergistic muscles of each exercise, as revealed on ExRx.net
- ensure that the number of exercises and sets prescribed for opposing muscles and opposing movement patterns generally agree with the ratios.

For example, since the strengths of your hip extensors and hip flexors should be equal, I tried to make sure that the number of exercises and sets that hit those muscles is approximately equal.

Note that balancing the Women's Beginner program wasn't as important as balancing the other programs because the Women's Beginner program isn't intended to be repeated over and over again and is designed to prepare you for the subsequent programs. Even so, it is still relatively balanced.

Exercises for curves

Generally speaking, curves are the product of having a high shoulders-to-waist ratio and a low waist-to-hips ratio, producing the desired hourglass figure. In order to promote these ratios, I ensured that the MCFS and Women's Plateau Buster programs include an appropriate balance of exercises for shoulders, hips, inner and outer thighs, and especially glutes. Balancing these kinds of programs leads to complications, which I'd like to briefly share.

One of the complications is that many exercises that are great for glutes, such as the squat and lunge, are also great for quadriceps. Since most women don't want big quadriceps, I prescribed variations of these exercises that emphasize glutes and hamstrings over quadriceps (such as the sumo squat and the forward-leaning lunge). All the while, I had to maintain the recommended quadriceps–hamstrings balance.

Another problem encountered when designing programs for curves is that the relatively large number of glute exercises have to be balanced with hip flexor exercises because the hip flexors are the opposing muscle group. The issue is that beginners with a weak rectus abdominis who perform lots of hip flexion exercises using improper form can develop lower back problems because the rectus abdominis can't counter the hip flexors' pull on the lumbar spine. Therefore, I had to make sure that the Women's Beginner mesocycle started by strengthening the rectus abdominis a little, before gradually easing hip flexion into the mix. Then, of course, I had to balance the ab exercises with exercises for the erector spinae, which oppose the abs and should ideally be equally as strong.

Exercises for functional strength

Functional strength is the kind of strength that is useful outside of the gym, in everyday activities. You develop functional strength by strengthening the ways in which your body is designed to move. The ways in which your body is designed to move can be broken down into seven "primal" movement patterns:

1. Squatting
2. Lunging (forward, sideways, or backward)
3. Flexing/Extending the hips
4. Pushing (horizontally or vertically)
5. Pulling (horizontally or vertically)
6. Twisting (or resisting twisting forces)
7. Walking/Running (gait)

You use these primal movement patterns in various combinations every day of your life. By strengthening them, you not only develop a functionally strong body but also:

- enhance your motor control, coordination, balance, and flexibility
- become better equipped for everyday activities
- improve your overall fitness and athleticism.

Unfortunately, most training programs that you encounter do not cover these movement patterns. Instead, they focus on training muscles, often in isolation, which is not how the body is designed to work. Rest assured that the weight training programs in this book, together with the FCT cardio program, incorporate effective functional training and give you the benefits outlined above.

Exercises for strengthening the core

An important element of having a functionally strong body is to have a strong core. Your core isn't just your rectus abdominis and lower back; it's your entire torso, especially all of the deep muscles that attach to your spinal column and pelvis. Your core muscles help to:

- stabilize your body when you lift
- transfer weight from one side of your body to the other
- transfer weight from your lower body to your upper body.

Your core is also where you generate much of your power. As such, it acts as your power base, power transfer center, and stabilization facility. Having a strong core is therefore of major importance for progress and overall fitness and athleticism.

Proper core training involves performing a range of major compound and functional exercises designed to strengthen both the deep and superficial muscles of the core, ideally, both dynamically and isometrically. All of the weight training programs in this book incorporate effective dynamic core training, while some also include isometric core training.

Summary of programming rules and objectives

When designing the weight training programs for women, I tried to follow or satisfy the following rules and objectives:

- Train all muscle groups at least twice a week
- Strengthen all primal movement patterns using compound and functional exercises
- Prescribe exercises and sets for opposing muscles and movement patterns in accordance with recommended muscle strength balance ratios
- Undulate rep ranges to simultaneously develop multiple muscle properties and maintain properties developed in previous mesocycles
- Strengthen the core using compound, functional, and unilateral exercises
- Train the core dynamically and isometrically
- Only include exercises the equipment for which should be available in any gym
- Incorporate exercise variation to maintain engagement
- Avoid exercises that have a high risk-to-benefit ratio, such as the narrow-grip upright row and behind-the-neck pulls and presses
- Favor free-weight exercises over machine exercises
- Avoid overworking the supraspinatus muscle, which is a common mistake
- Train large muscle groups before small muscle groups
- Prescribe more sets for large muscle groups than for small muscle groups
- Keep most workouts to approximately 18 or fewer sets, which produces workouts that last for approximately 50 minutes or less (the more advanced workouts include up to 21 sets)
- Force gradual but definite progress from mesocycle to mesocycle
- Ensure adequate rest by enforcing regular deload weeks

Alternative exercises

If you get bored of an exercise, or if you can't perform an exercise for some reason, you can swap it for one of the alternative exercises below without significantly affecting the balance of your program.

Legs and glutes

- Hyperextension – Straight-leg deadlift
- Romanian deadlift – Cable pull-through
- Squat – Front squat – Hack squat – Sumo squat – Zercher squat – Jefferson squat
- Forward/Rear/Side lunge – Step-up – Split squat –Bulgarian split squat
- Lying leg curl – Seated leg curl – Inverse leg curl
- Machine standing calf raise – Standing one-leg dumbbell calf raise – Leg-press calf press
- Barbell hip thrust – Barbell glute bridge

- Cable standing hip abduction – Machine seated hip abduction
- Cable standing hip adduction – Machine seated hip adduction

Back

- Lat pull-down – Pull-up (medium grip is best)
- Bent-over dumbbell row – Barbell row – T-bar row – Straight-back seated cable row – Inverted row
- Seated cable row – Wide-grip seated cable row

Chest

- Bench press – Push-up – Cable/Machine chest press

Shoulders

- Overhead press – Arnold press
- Cable face pull – Dumbbell face pull – Cuban rotation
- Lying dumbbell external shoulder rotation – Cable external shoulder rotation

Arms

- Triceps rope push-down – Dumbbell/Cable kickback – Triceps overhead extension – Lying triceps extension (French press) – Skull crusher
- Triceps dip – Bench dip – Diamond push-up – Close-grip bench press/push-up
- Dumbbell/Barbell curl – EZ bar curl (bar must have minimal camber)

Core

- Front plank – Ab walkout – Inch worm – Wheel rollout
- Cable wood chop – Weighted Russian twist – Weighted lying oblique twist
- Lying leg raise – Hanging leg raise – Captain's chair leg raise
- Lying straight leg raise – Hanging straight leg raise – Captain's chair straight leg raise – Stability ball pike
- Lying leg and hip raise – Hanging leg and hip raise – Captain's chair leg and hip raise

Women's Beginner

Description

The 12-week Women's Beginner program is designed to:

- introduce your body to physical exercise
- introduce you to a variety of exercises, training equipment, and training splits
- train all of your major muscle groups

- strengthen your core and primal movement patterns
- encourage body-wide neuromuscular adaptation
- promote the development of a strong foundation of muscular endurance upon which you can safely build in the subsequent programs. Without this strong foundation, you will be at risk of injury.

By the end of the program, you should have:

- developed significant strength (mostly due to neuromuscular adaptation), muscular endurance, and muscular "tone"
- dramatically improved your overall fitness.

The Women's Beginner program is divided into four sections (microcycles), each one lasting for three weeks. The first two microcycles focus on full-body circuit training, which means that you will be training your entire body in each workout. The last two microcycles focus on split training, which means that you will be dividing your body into sections and training them in separate workouts.

Please don't be intimidated by the number of exercises in some of the workouts. You will be flying through them with minimal rest, so the workouts will be completed very quickly.

Please read the **Overview of women's training programs**, at the beginning of this chapter, before starting this program.

Suitability

- Beginners
- Individuals who have less than 3 months of consistent weight training experience
- Experienced individuals who haven't trained for more than 3 months

General instructions

- Complete the exercises in the order presented.
- Always use a weight that's heavy enough to make the reps challenging.
- Whenever you have to increase the weight, add a maximum of 5 lb (2.5 kg) to upper-body exercises or a maximum of 10 lb (5 kg) to lower-body exercises.
- Try to master the proper form of each exercise, including proper breathing technique. Instructions for most exercises are available on my website, **weighttraining.guide**. Also, try to develop a mental connection with your muscles and with the movement patterns.
- If training at home in the absence of cable machines and other specialized equipment, see below the exercise tables for exercise alternatives.
- Don't forget to warm up before, and cool down after, each workout.
- Once you have completed the Women's Beginner program, you must take a deload week (a week during which you either rest or train lightly). Only then can you move on to the next program.

Specific instructions for each microcycle are presented below.

Microcycle 1: Full-body circuit (3 weeks)

- For microcycle 1, you will perform a full-body circuit.
- Complete 3 workouts per week, with at least 1 day of rest between each workout (e.g. AXAXAXX, where "A" is a workout day and "X" is a rest day).
- Complete 2 circuits per workout.
- Rest for only 20–30 seconds between exercises.
- Rest for 2–3 minutes before starting the second circuit.
- Each workout should take less than 30 minutes.

Exercise	Reps
Dumbbell sumo squat*	15–18
Medium-grip lat pull-down	15–18
Hyperextension	15–18
Dumbbell bench press	15–18
Seated or lying leg curl	15–18
Straight-back seated cable row	15–18
Machine standing calf raise	25–30
Seated dumbbell overhead press	15–18
Bicycle crunch	15–20
*Bodyweight squat for first week	

Alternatives for cable/machine exercises

- Medium-grip lat pull-down — Medium-grip band lat pull-down or medium-grip self-assisted pull-up
- Hyperextension — Straight-leg deadlift
- Seated or lying leg curl — Inverse leg curl, stability ball leg curl, or band leg curl
- Straight-back seated cable row — Bent-over dumbbell row or straight-back band row
- Machine standing calf raise — Standing dumbbell one-leg calf raise or band standing calf raise

Microcycle 2: Full-body circuit (3 weeks)

- For microcycle 2, you will perform a more comprehensive full-body circuit.
- Complete either 3 workouts a week (AXAXAXX) or a workout every other day (AX).
- Complete 2 circuits per workout.
- Rest for only 20–30 seconds between exercises.
- Rest for 2–3 minutes before starting the second circuit.
- Each workout should take less than 40 minutes.

Exercise	Reps
Barbell squat (wear loop band around thighs if available)	13–15
Medium-grip lat pull-down	13–15
Dumbbell Romanian deadlift	13–15
Push-up on knees or on stability ball	13–15
Weighted one-leg hip thrust	13–15
Bent-over dumbbell row	13–15
Seated or lying leg curl	13–15
Dumbbell one-arm overhead press	13–15
Lying alternating straight leg raise	15–20
Dumbbell curl	13–15
Standing dumbbell one-leg calf raise	25–30
Bicycle crunch	20–25

Alternatives for cable/machine exercises

- Medium-grip lat pull-down — Medium-grip band lat pull-down or medium-grip self-assisted pull-up
- Seated or lying leg curl — Inverse leg curl, stability ball leg curl, or band leg curl

Microcycle 3: Upper–Lower split (3 weeks)

- For microcycle 3, you will perform an upper–lower split. This means that you will train all of your upper body in one workout (Workout A) and all of your lower body in another workout (Workout

B). Also, instead of circuit training, you will perform set training, which means that you will complete all of the sets for one exercise before moving on to the sets of the following exercise.

- The recommended workout schedules are ABXABXX or ABX.
- Rest for only 20–30 seconds between sets.
- Rest for only 60–90 seconds between exercises.
- Each workout should take less than 40 minutes.

Workout A (Upper Body)	
Exercise	Sets x Reps
Seated cable row	2 x 13–15
One-arm lat pull-down	2 x 13–15
Push-up on knees or on stability ball	2 x 13–15
Barbell overhead press	2 x 13–15
Cable face pull	2 x 13–15
Triceps rope push-down	2 x 13–15
EZ bar curl	2 x 13–15
Cable twist	2 x 13–15
Front plank	2 x 45–60 s
s = seconds	

Workout B (Lower Body)	
Exercise	Sets x Reps
Barbell front squat (wear loop band around thighs if available)	2 x 13–15
Dumbbell lunge	2 x 13–15
Barbell Romanian deadlift	2 x 13–15
Barbell hip thrust	2 x 13–15
Seated or lying leg curl	2 x 13–15
Lying leg and hip raise	2 x 15–20
Bicycle crunch	2 x 20–25
Lying alternating straight leg raise	2 x 20–25
Standing dumbbell one-leg calf raise	2 x 20–25

Alternatives for cable/machine exercises

- Seated cable row — Bent-over dumbbell row, bent-over barbell row, or band row
- One-arm lat pull-down — One-arm band lat pull-down or self-assisted pull-up
- Cable face pull — Dumbbell face pull or band face pull
- Triceps rope push-down — Dumbbell kickback or triceps band push-down
- Cable twist — Weighted Russian twist or band twist
- Seated or lying leg curl — Inverse leg curl, one-leg stability ball leg curl, or band leg curl

Microcycle 4: 3-day split (3 weeks)

- For microcycle 4, you will perform a 3-day split in which you will train your back, biceps, and core in Workout A; your chest, shoulders, triceps, and core in Workout B; and your legs and glutes in Workout C.
- The recommended workout schedules are ABCXABX (then start from C the next week) or ABCX (i.e. three days on, one day off).
- Rest for only 20–30 seconds between sets.
- Rest for only 60–90 seconds between exercises.
- Each workout should take less than 40 minutes.

Workout A (Back, biceps, core)	
Exercise	Sets x Reps
Barbell sumo deadlift	2 x 12–14
Machine-assisted pull-up	2 x 12–14
Cable twisting one-arm row	2 x 12–14
Dumbbell curl	2 x 12–14
Dumbbell side bend	2 x 15–20
Lying side hip raise	2 x 15–20
Bicycle crunch	2 x 25–30
Wheel rollout	2 x 10–15

Workout B (Chest, shoulders, triceps, core)	
Exercise	**Sets x Reps**
Standing cable chest press	2 x 12–14
Dumbbell one-arm overhead press	2 x 12–14
Dumbbell bent-over lateral raise	2 x 12–14
Cable face pull	2 x 12–14
Diamond push-up on knees	2 x 12–14
Cable wood chop	2 x 12–14
Captain's chair leg and hip raise	2 x 12–14
Lying alternating straight leg raise	2 x 25–30

Workout C (Legs, glutes)	
Exercise	**Sets x Reps**
Barbell sumo squat	2 x 12–14
Dumbbell Bulgarian split squat	2 x 12–14
Weighted one-leg hip thrust	2 x 12–14
Smith machine kneeling rear kick	2 x 12–14
Seated or lying leg curl	2 x 12–14
Cable hip abduction	2 x 15–20
Cable hip adduction	2 x 15–20
Machine standing calf raise	2 x 20–25

Alternatives for cable/machine exercises

- Machine-assisted pull-up — Self-assisted pull-up or band lat pull-down
- Cable twisting one-arm row — Band twisting one-arm row or dumbbell twisting row
- Wheel rollout — Ab walkout or inch worm
- Standing cable chest press — Bench press or standing band chest press
- Cable face pull — Dumbbell face pull or band face pull
- Cable wood chop — Band wood chop or weighted Russian twist
- Captain's chair leg and hip raise — Lying or hanging leg and hip raise
- Smith machine kneeling rear kick — Band rear kick or one-leg glute bridge

- Seated or lying leg curl — Inverse leg curl, one-leg stability ball leg curl, or band leg curl
- Cable hip abduction — Band hip abduction or side plank hip abduction
- Cable hip adduction — Band hip adduction or side plank hip adduction
- Machine standing calf raise — Standing dumbbell one-leg calf raise or band standing calf raise

Maximum Curves and Functional Strength 1

Description

The 8-week Maximum Curves and Functional Strength 1 program is designed to:

- train all of your major muscle groups
- build muscle/curves in the 9–11 rep range
- strengthen your core and primal movement patterns
- introduce you to the intensity technique of superset training.

The program is a three-day training split, which means that you will divide your body into three and train each of the three sections in a separate workout. In Workout A, you will train your back, biceps, and core; in Workout B, you will train your chest, shoulders, triceps, and core; and in Workout C, you will train your legs and glutes.

Since you are training in the 9–11 rep range and therefore using heavier weights than you used in the Women's Beginner program, you will be resting a little longer between sets and exercises.

Please read the **Overview of women's training programs**, at the beginning of this chapter, before you start this program.

Suitability

- Individuals who have completed the Women's Beginner program
- Anyone who has at least 3 months of consistent weight training experience

Instructions

- Complete the workouts (A, B, and C) in the order presented.
- The recommend workout schedules are ABCX (i.e. three days on, one day off) or ABCXABX (i.e. three days on, one day off, two days on, one day off, and then continue the sequence from where you left off).
- Complete all of the sets for one exercise before moving on to the sets of the following exercise.
- Rest for 30–90 seconds between sets.
- Rest for 1–2 minutes between exercises.
- Always use an amount of weight that makes completing the reps challenging.

- Whenever you have to increase the weight, add a maximum of 5 lb (2.5 kg) to upper-body exercises or a maximum of 10 lb (5 kg) to lower-body exercises.
- Try to master the proper form of each exercise, including proper breathing technique. Instructions for most exercises are available on my website, **weighttraining.guide**. Also, try to develop a mental connection with your muscles and with the movement patterns.
- If you get bored of an exercise, see the **Overview of women's training programs** for alternatives.
- If training at home in the absence of cable machines and other specialized equipment, see below the exercise tables for exercise alternatives.
- If possible, perform the exercises marked with an asterisk (*) as a superset (i.e. after you perform a set of one exercise, perform a set of the other exercise without resting).
- Don't forget to warm up before, and cool down after, each workout.
- Once you have completed Maximum Curves and Functional Strength 1, you must take a deload week. Only then can you move on to the next program or repeat the same program.

Workout A (Back, biceps, core)	
Exercise	**Sets x Reps**
Barbell deadlift	3 x 9–11
Machine-assisted pull-up	2 x 9–11
Seated cable row	3 x 9–11
EZ bar curl*	2 x 9–11
Lying side hip raise*	3 x 20–25
Bicycle crunch	3 x 20–25
*To be performed as a superset	

Workout B (Chest, shoulders, triceps, core)	
Exercise	**Sets x Reps**
Push-up (on knees if necessary)	3 x 9–11
Barbell overhead press	2 x 9–11
Barbell wide-grip upright row	2 x 9–11
Cable face pull	3 x 9–11
Weighted bench dip*	2 x 9–11
Cable down-up twist*	2 x 9–11

172

Wheel rollout	3 x 10–15
*To be performed as a superset	

Workout C (Legs, glutes)	
Exercise	**Sets x Reps**
Barbell sumo squat	3 x 9–11
Dumbbell forward-leaning lunge	2 x 9–11
Seated or lying leg curl	3 x 9–11
Barbell hip thrust	2 x 9–11
Cable hip abduction	2 x 15–20
Standing dumbbell one-leg calf raise*	3 x 15–20
Captain's chair leg and hip raise with dumbbell between feet*	3 x 9–11
*To be performed as a superset	

Alternatives for cable/machine exercises

- Machine-assisted pull-up — Self-assisted pull-up or band lat pull-down
- Seated cable row — Bent-over dumbbell row, bent-over barbell row, or band row
- Cable face pull — Dumbbell face pull or band face pull
- Cable down-up twist — Band down-up twist or weighted Russian twist
- Wheel rollout — Ab walkout or inch worm
- Seated or lying leg curl — Inverse leg curl, one-leg stability ball leg curl, or band leg curl
- Cable hip abduction — Band hip abduction or side plank hip abduction
- Captain's chair leg and hip raise with dumbbell between feet — Hanging leg and hip raise with dumbbell between feet or lying leg and hip raise with bands attached to ankles

Maximum Curves and Functional Strength 2

Description

The 10-week Maximum Curves and Functional Strength 2 program is designed to:

- train all of your major muscle groups

- build muscle/curves in the 9–11 and 6–8 rep ranges
- strengthen your core and primal movement patterns
- introduce you to rep-range alternation (undulating periodization)
- introduce you to the intensity technique of training to failure.

The program consists of two upper–lower splits, which means that there are four workouts per week, two for your upper body (A and C) and two for your lower body (B and D).

In weeks 1, 3, 5, 7, and 9, you will train in the 9–11 rep range; in weeks 2, 4, 6, 8, and 10, you will train in the 6–8 rep range.

Please read the **Overview of women's training programs**, at the beginning of this chapter, to understand why you will be alternating rep ranges.

Suitability

- Individuals who have completed Maximum Curves and Functional Strength 1
- Anyone who has at least 6 months of consistent weight training experience

Instructions

- Complete the workouts (A, B, C, and D) in the order provided.
- The recommend schedule is ABXCDXX (where "X" is a rest day). Avoid training four days on, three days off (i.e. ABCDXXX).
- Rest for 30–90 seconds between sets.
- Rest for 1–2 minutes between exercises.
- Always use a weight that is heavy enough to make the reps challenging.
- Whenever you have to increase the weight, add a maximum of 5 lb (2.5 kg) to upper-body exercises or a maximum of 10 lb (5 kg) to lower-body exercises.
- Try to master the proper form of each exercise, including proper breathing technique. Instructions for most exercises are available on my website, **weighttraining.guide**. Also, try to develop a mental connection with your muscles and with the movement patterns.
- If you get bored of an exercise, see the **Overview of women's training programs** for alternatives.
- If training at home in the absence of cable machines and other specialized equipment, see below the exercise tables for exercise alternatives.
- In weeks 1, 3, 5, 7, and 9, take the last set of every exercise to failure — that is, keep doing reps until you can't do another rep in good form. This is an intensity technique known as training to failure. Note that for some exercises, such as the barbell squat, you will not be able to safely train to failure unless you have a training partner ready, in which case you should not train to failure.
- Don't forget to warm up before, and cool down after, each workout.
- Once you have completed Maximum Curves and Functional Strength 2, you must take a deload week. Only then can you move on to the next program or repeat the same program.

174

Workout A (Upper Body)		
Exercise	Sets x Reps	
	*Weeks 1, 3, 5, 7, 9	Weeks 2, 4, 6, 8, 10
Medium-grip lat pull-down	3 x 9–11	3 x 6–8
Cable chest press	3 x 9–11	3 x 6–8
Seated dumbbell overhead press	2 x 9–11	2 x 6–8
Cable face pull	3 x 9–11	3 x 6–8
Triceps rope push-down	2 x 9–11	2 x 6–8
EZ bar curl	3 x 9–11	3 x 6–8
Front plank	2 x 60–90 s	2 x 90–120 s
*If possible, take the last set of every exercise to failure. s = seconds		

Workout B (Lower Body)		
Exercise	Sets x Reps	
	*Weeks 1, 3, 5, 7, 9	Weeks 2, 4, 6, 8, 10
Barbell sumo squat	3 x 9–11	3 x 6–8
Barbell or weighted one-leg hip thrust	2 x 9–11	2 x 6–8
Seated or lying leg curl	2 x 9–11	2 x 6–8
Smith machine kneeling rear kick	2 x 9–11	2 x 6–8
Lying side hip raise	2 x 20–25	2 x 25–30
Bicycle crunch	3 x 20–25	3 x 25–30
Standing dumbbell one-leg calf raise	3 x 15–20	3 x 10–15
*If possible, take the last set of every exercise to failure		

Workout C (Upper Body)		
Exercise	Sets x Reps	
	*Weeks 1, 3, 5, 7, 9	Weeks 2, 4, 6, 8, 10
Cable twisting one-arm row	3 x 9–11	3 x 6–8

Push-up (on stability ball if available)	3 x 9–11	3 x 12–14
Dumbbell bent-over lateral raise	2 x 9–11	2 x 6–8
Dumbbell lying external shoulder rotation	2 x 15–20	2 x 10–15
Triceps dip with dumbbell between feet	2 x 9–11	2 x 6–8
Dumbbell curl	3 x 9–11	3 x 6–8
Wheel rollout	3 x 10–15	3 x 15–20
*If possible, take the last set of every exercise to failure		

Workout D (Lower Body)		
	Sets x Reps	
Exercise	*Weeks 1, 3, 5, 7, 9	Weeks 2, 4, 6, 8, 10
Barbell Romanian deadlift	3 x 9–11	3 x 6–8
Barbell Bulgarian split squat	2 x 9–11	2 x 6–8
Seated or lying leg curl	2 x 9–11	2 x 6–8
Cable hip abduction	2 x 15–20	2 x 10–15
Cable wood chop	2 x 9–11	2 x 6–8
Captain's chair leg and hip raise with dumbbell between feet	3 x 9–11	3 x 6–8
Machine standing calf raise	3 x 15–20	3 x 10–15
*If possible, take the last set of every exercise to failure		

Alternatives for cable/machine exercises

- Medium-grip lat pull-down — Medium-grip band lat pull-down or medium-grip self-assisted pull-up
- Cable chest press — Band chest press or dumbbell bench press
- Cable face pull — Dumbbell face pull or band face pull
- Triceps rope push-down — Dumbbell kickback or triceps band push-down
- Seated or lying leg curl — Inverse leg curl, one-leg stability ball leg curl, or band leg curl
- Smith machine kneeling rear kick — Band rear kick or barbell one-leg glute bridge
- Cable twisting one-arm row — Band twisting one-arm row or dumbbell twisting row
- Triceps dip — Weighted bench dip
- Wheel rollout — Ab walkout or inch worm
- Cable hip abduction — Band hip abduction or side plank hip abduction

- Cable wood chop — Band wood chop or weighted Russian twist
- Captain's chair leg and hip raise with dumbbell between feet — Hanging leg and hip raise with dumbbell between feet or lying leg and hip raise with bands attached to ankles
- Machine standing calf raise — Standing dumbbell one-leg calf raise or band standing calf raise

Maximum Curves and Functional Strength 3

Description

The 10-week Maximum Curves and Functional Strength 3 program is designed to:

- train all of your major muscle groups
- build muscle/curves in the 9–11 and 6–8 rep ranges
- strengthen your core and primal movement patterns
- introduce you to the dropset intensity training technique.

The program consists of two push–pull splits, which means that there are four workouts per week, two for your push muscles (A and C) and two for your pull muscles (B and D).

In weeks 1, 3, 5, 7, and 9, you will train in the 9–11 rep range; in weeks 2, 4, 6, 8, and 10, you will train in the 6–8 rep range.

Please read the **Overview of women's training programs**, at the beginning of this chapter, before you start this program.

Suitability

- Individuals who have completed Maximum Curves and Functional Strength 2
- Anyone who has at least 6 months of consistent weight training experience

Instructions

- Complete the workouts (A, B, C, and D) in the order provided.
- The recommend schedule is ABXCDXX (where "X" is a rest day). Avoid training four days on and three days off (i.e. ABCDXXX).
- Rest for 30–90 seconds between sets.
- Rest for 1–2 minutes between exercises.
- Always use an amount of weight that makes completing the reps challenging.
- Whenever you have to increase the weight, add a maximum of 5 lb (2.5 kg) to upper-body exercises or a maximum of 10 lb (5 kg) to lower-body exercises.

- Try to master the proper form of each exercise, including proper breathing technique. Instructions for most exercises are available on my website, **weighttraining.guide**. Also, try to develop a mental connection with your muscles and with the movement patterns.
- If you get bored of an exercise, see the **Overview of women's training programs** for alternatives.
- If training at home in the absence of cable machines and other specialized equipment, see below the exercise tables for exercise alternatives.
- In weeks 1, 3, 5, 7, and 9, take the last set of every exercise to failure. Then, without resting, reduce the amount of weight on the bar and continue until failure again. This intensity technique is known as dropset training. Note that it is not safe to use it on some exercises, such as the barbell squat, unless you have a spotter. Therefore, if you do not have a spotter, do not use the technique on these exercises.
- Don't forget to warm up before, and cool down after, each workout.
- Once you have completed Maximum Curves and Functional Strength 3, you must take a deload week. Only then can you move on to the next program or repeat the same program.

Workout A (Pull)		
Exercise	**Sets x Reps**	
	***Weeks 1, 3, 5, 7, 9**	**Weeks 2, 4, 6, 8, 10**
Barbell deadlift	3 x 9–11	3 x 6–8
Seated or lying leg curl	2 x 9–11	2 x 6–8
Cable twisting one-arm row	3 x 9–11	3 x 6–8
Dumbbell bent-over lateral raise	2 x 9–11	2 x 6–8
Incline dumbbell curl	2 x 9–11	2 x 6–8
Captain's chair leg and hip raise with dumbbell between feet	3 x 9–11	3 x 6–8
Wheel rollout	3 x 10–15	3 x 15–20
*If possible, perform a dropset for the last set of every exercise		

Workout B (Push)		
Exercise	**Sets x Reps**	
	***Weeks 1, 3, 5, 7, 9**	**Weeks 2, 4, 6, 8, 10**
Dumbbell rear lunge	3 x 9–11	3 x 6–8
Barbell hip thrust	2 x 9–11	2 x 6–8

Exercise	Weeks 1, 3, 5, 7, 9	Weeks 2, 4, 6, 8, 10
Standing dumbbell one-leg calf raise	3 x 15–20	3 x 10–15
Barbell bench press	3 x 9–11	3 x 6–8
Diamond push-up (on knees if necessary)	2 x 9–11	2 x 12–14
Lying side hip raise	2 x 20–25	2 x 25–30
One-leg front plank	2 x 60–90 s	2 x 90–120 s

*If possible, perform a dropset for the last set of every exercise. s = seconds.

Workout C (Pull)		
	Sets x Reps	
Exercise	*Weeks 1, 3, 5, 7, 9	Weeks 2, 4, 6, 8, 10
Weighted inverted row	3 x 9–11	3 x 6–8
One-arm lat pull-down	3 x 9–11	3 x 6–8
Cable face pull	3 x 9–11	3 x 6–8
EZ bar curl	2 x 9–11	2 x 6–8
Twisting hyperextension holding a plate against chest	2 x 9–11	2 x 6–8
Bicycle crunch	3 x 20–25	3 x 25–30
Lying straight leg raise	2 x 20–25	2 x 25–30

*If possible, perform a dropset for the last set of every exercise

Workout D (Push)		
	Sets x Reps	
Exercise	*Weeks 1, 3, 5, 7, 9	Weeks 2, 4, 6, 8, 10
Barbell sumo squat	3 x 9–11	3 x 6–8
Smith machine kneeling rear kick	2 x 9–11	2 x 6–8
Cable hip abduction	2 x 15–20	2 x 10–15
Machine standing calf raise	3 x 15–20	3 x 10–15
Push-up (on stability ball if available)	3 x 9–11	3 x 12–14
Dumbbell one-arm overhead press	2 x 9–11	2 x 6–8

Triceps dip with dumbbell between feet	2 x 9–11	2 x 6–8
*If possible, perform a dropset for the last set of every exercise		

Alternatives for cable/machine exercises

- Seated or lying leg curl — Inverse leg curl, one-leg stability ball leg curl, or band leg curl
- Cable twisting one-arm row — Band twisting one-arm row or dumbbell twisting row
- Captain's chair leg and hip raise with dumbbell between feet — Hanging leg and hip raise with dumbbell between feet or lying leg and hip raise with bands attached to ankles
- Wheel rollout — Ab walkout or inch worm
- Weighted inverted row — Bent-over barbell row or seated band row
- One-arm lat pull-down — One-arm band lat pull-down, self-assisted pull-up, or pull-up
- Cable face pull — Dumbbell face pull or band face pull
- Twisting hyperextension holding a plate against chest — Twisting hyperextension on flat bench holding a plate against chest
- Smith machine kneeling rear kick — Band rear kick or barbell one-leg glute bridge
- Cable hip abduction — Band hip abduction or side plank hip abduction
- Machine standing calf raise — Standing dumbbell one-leg calf raise or band standing calf raise
- Triceps dip — Weighted bench dip

Maximum Curves and Functional Strength 4

Description

The 8-week Maximum Curves and Functional Strength 4 program is designed to:

- train all of your major muscle groups
- build muscle/curves in the 9–11 and 6–8 rep ranges
- strengthen your core and primal movement patterns
- introduce you to the rest–pause intensity training technique.

The program consists of five workouts (A, B, C, D, and E). Workout A will train your back, biceps, and core; Workout B will train your chest, shoulders, triceps, and core; Workout C will train your legs, glutes, and core; Workout D will train your upper body; and Workout E will train your lower body.

In weeks 1, 3, 5, and 7, you will train in the 9–11 rep range; in weeks 2, 4, 6, and 8, you will train in the 6–8 rep range.

Please read the **Overview of women's training programs**, at the beginning of this chapter, before you start this program.

Suitability

- Individuals who have completed Maximum Curves and Functional Strength 3
- Anyone who has at least 9 months of consistent weight training experience

Instructions

- Complete the workouts in the order presented.
- The recommend workout schedule is ABCXDEX (where "X" is a rest day). Avoid training five days on and two days off (i.e. ABCDEXX).
- Rest for 30–90 seconds between sets.
- Rest for 1–2 minutes between exercises.
- Always use a weight that is heavy enough to make the reps challenging.
- Whenever you have to increase the weight, add a maximum of 5 lb (2.5 kg) to upper-body exercises or a maximum of 10 lb (5 kg) to lower-body exercises.
- Try to master the proper form of each exercise, including proper breathing technique. Instructions for most exercises are available on my website, **weighttraining.guide**. Also, try to develop a mental connection with your muscles and with the movement patterns.
- If you get bored of an exercise, see the **Overview of women's training programs** for alternatives.
- If training at home in the absence of cable machines and other specialized equipment, see below the exercise tables for exercise alternatives.
- In weeks 1, 3, 5, and 7, take the last set of every exercise to failure, put down the weights, wait for 15–20 seconds, pick the weights back up, and continue until you hit failure again. This intensity technique is known as rest–pause training. Note that it's unsafe to use it on some exercises, such as the barbell squat, unless you have a spotter ready. Therefore, if you do not have a spotter, do not use the technique on these exercises.
- Don't forget to warm up before, and cool down after, each workout.
- Once you have completed Maximum Curves and Functional Strength 4, you must take a deload week. Only then can you repeat the program or move on to the next program.

Workout A (Back, biceps, core)		
Exercise	**Sets x Reps**	
	*Weeks 1, 3, 5, 7	**Weeks 2, 4, 6, 8**
Machine-assisted pull-up	3 x 9–11	3 x 6–8
Seated cable row	3 x 9–11	3 x 6–8
EZ bar curl	2 x 9–11	2 x 6–8
Dumbbell lying external shoulder rotation	2 x 15–20	2 x 10–15
Bicycle crunch	3 x 20–25	3 x 25–30

| Lying side hip raise | 3 x 20–25 | 3 x 25–30 |

*If possible, perform a rest pause for the last set of every exercise

Workout B (Chest, shoulders, triceps, core)		
Exercise	**Sets x Reps**	
	*Weeks 1, 3, 5, 7	**Weeks 2, 4, 6, 8**
Push-up	3 x 9–11	3 x 12–14
Barbell overhead press	3 x 9–11	3 x 6–8
Dumbbell lateral raise	2 x 9–11	2 x 6–8
Cable face pull	3 x 9–11	3 x 6–8
One-arm bench dip	2 x 9–11	2 x 12–14
Cable twist	2 x 9–11	2 x 6–8
Wheel rollout	3 x 10–15	3 x 15–20

*If possible, perform a rest pause for the last set of every exercise

Workout C (Legs, glutes, core)		
Exercise	**Sets x Reps**	
	*Weeks 1, 3, 5, 7	**Weeks 2, 4, 6, 8**
Barbell sumo squat	3 x 9–11	3 x 6–8
One-leg hyperextension holding a plate against chest	2 x 9–11	2 x 6–8
Smith machine kneeling rear kick	2 x 9–11	2 x 6–8
Seated or lying leg curl	3 x 9–11	3 x 6–8
Lying alternating straight leg raise	2 x 25–30	2 x 30–35
One-leg front plank	2 x 60–90 s	2 x 90–120 s
Machine standing calf raise	3 x 15–20	3 x 10–15

*If possible, perform a rest pause for the last set of every exercise. s = seconds

Workout D (Upper Body)		
Exercise	**Sets x Reps**	
	*Weeks 1, 3, 5, 7	Weeks 2, 4, 6, 8
Weighted inverted row	3 x 9–11	3 x 6–8
One-arm lat pull-down	2 x 9–11	2 x 6–8
Cable chest press	3 x 9–11	3 x 6–8
Diamond push-up (on knees if necessary)	2 x 9–11	2 x 12–14
Dumbbell bent-over lateral raise	3 x 9–11	3 x 6–8
Triceps rope push-down	2 x 9–11	2 x 6–8
Dumbbell curl	2 x 9–11	2 x 6–8
*If possible, perform a rest pause for the last set of every exercise		

Workout E (Lower Body)		
Exercise	**Sets x Reps**	
	*Weeks 1, 3, 5, 7	Weeks 2, 4, 6, 8
Barbell deadlift	3 x 9–11	3 x 6–8
Dumbbell forward-leaning lunge	2 x 9–11	2 x 6–8
Barbell hip thrust	2 x 9–11	2 x 6–8
Cable hip abduction	2 x 15–20	2 x 10–15
Cable hip adduction	2 x 15–20	2 x 10–15
Captain's chair leg and hip raise with dumbbell between feet	3 x 9–11	3 x 6–8
Machine seated one-leg calf raise	3 x 15–20	3 x 10–15
*If possible, perform a rest pause for the last set of every exercise		

Alternatives for cable/machine exercises

- Machine-assisted pull-up — Self-assisted pull-up or band lat pull-down
- Seated cable row — Bent-over dumbbell row, bent-over barbell row, or band row
- Cable face pull — Dumbbell face pull or band face pull
- Cable twist — Weighted Russian twist or band twist
- Wheel rollout — Ab walkout or inch worm

- One-leg hyperextension holding a plate against chest — One-leg straight-leg deadlift
- Smith machine kneeling rear kick — Band rear kick or barbell one-leg glute bridge
- Seated or lying leg curl — Inverse leg curl, one-leg stability ball leg curl, or band leg curl
- Machine standing calf raise — Standing dumbbell one-leg calf raise or band standing calf raise
- Weighted inverted row — Bent-over barbell row or seated band row
- One-arm lat pull-down — One-arm band lat pull-down, self-assisted pull-up, or pull-up
- Cable chest press — Band chest press or dumbbell bench press
- Triceps rope push-down — Skull crusher or triceps band push-down
- Cable hip abduction — Band hip abduction or side plank hip abduction
- Cable hip adduction — Band hip adduction or side plank hip adduction
- Captain's chair leg and hip raise with dumbbell between feet — Hanging leg and hip raise with dumbbell between feet or lying leg and hip raise with bands attached to ankles
- Machine seated one-leg calf raise — Barbell seated calf raise

Maximum Curves and Functional Strength 5

Description

The 12-week Maximum Curves and Functional Strength 5 program is designed to:

- train all of your major muscle groups
- build muscle/curves in the 9–11 and 6–8 rep ranges
- strengthen your core and primal movement patterns
- increase training intensity and volume (the number of exercises and sets that you perform) while reducing the amount of time that you spend in the gym.

The program consists of four workouts (A, B, C, and D). Workouts A and C will train your upper body and core; workouts B and D will train your lower body and core.

The exercises in all of the workouts have been arranged into supersets, which makes the workouts both shorter and more intense than the workouts of preceding programs.

In weeks 1, 3, 5, 7, 9, and 11, you will train in the 9–11 rep range; in weeks 2, 4, 6, 8, 10, and 12, you will train in the 6–8 rep range.

Please read the **Overview of women's training programs**, at the beginning of this chapter, before you start this program.

Suitability

- Individuals who have completed Maximum Curves and Functional Strength 4
- Anyone who has at least 12 months of consistent weight training experience

Instructions

- Complete the workouts in the order presented.
- The recommend workout schedule is ABXCDXX (where "X" is a rest day). Try not to train four days on and three days off (i.e. ABCDXXX).
- The exercises are arranged into pairs as supersets. After you complete one set of the first exercise, perform a set of the second exercise without resting.
- Rest for 1 to 2 minutes before repeating the superset and before moving on to the next superset.
- Always use a weight that is heavy enough to make the reps challenging.
- Whenever you have to increase the weight, add a maximum of 5 lb (2.5 kg) to upper-body exercises or a maximum of 10 lb (5 kg) to lower-body exercises.
- Try to master the proper form of each exercise, including proper breathing technique. Instructions for most exercises are available on my website, **weighttraining.guide**. Also, try to develop a mental connection with your muscles and with the movement patterns.
- If you get bored of an exercise, see the **Overview of women's training programs** for alternatives.
- If training at home in the absence of cable machines and other specialized equipment, see below the exercise tables for exercise alternatives.
- Don't forget to warm up before, and cool down after, each workout.
- Once you have completed Maximum Curves and Functional Strength 5, you must take a deload week. Only then can you repeat the program or one of the other programs.

Workout A (Upper body and core)		
Exercise	**Sets x Reps**	
	Weeks 1, 3, 5, 7, 9, 11	**Weeks 2, 4, 6, 8, 10, 12**
Inverted row	2 x 10–15	2 x 15–20
Push-up (on knees if necessary)	2 x 10–15	2 x 15–20
Medium-grip lat pull-down	2 x 9–11	2 x 6–8
Dumbbell one-arm overhead press	2 x 9–11	2 x 6–8
Dumbbell lateral raise	2 x 9–11	2 x 6–8
Cable face pull	2 x 9–11	2 x 6–8
Dumbbell curl	2 x 9–11	2 x 6–8
Overhead barbell triceps extension	2 x 9–11	2 x 6–8
One-leg front plank	2 x 60–90 s	2 x 90–120 s
Lying side hip raise	2 x 20–25	2 x 25–30
s = seconds		

Workout B (Lower body and core)		
Exercise	**Sets x Reps**	
	Weeks 1, 3, 5, 7, 9, 11	**Weeks 2, 4, 6, 8, 10, 12**
Barbell sumo squat	2 x 9–11	2 x 6–8
Dumbbell Romanian deadlift	2 x 9–11	2 x 6–8
Dumbbell forward-leaning lunge	2 x 9–11	2 x 6–8
Bicycle crunch	2 x 20–25	2 x 25–30
Barbell hip thrust	2 x 9–11	2 x 6–8
Captain's chair leg and hip raise with dumbbell between feet	2 x 9–11	2 x 6–8
Machine standing calf raise	2 x 15–20	2 x 10–15
Wheel rollout	2 x 10–15	2 x 15–20
Hyperextension holding a plate against chest	2 x 9–11	2 x 6–8
Lying alternating straight leg raise	2 x 25–30	2 x 30–35

Workout C (Upper body and core)		
Exercise	**Sets x Reps**	
	Weeks 1, 3, 5, 7, 9, 11	**Weeks 2, 4, 6, 8, 10, 12**
Seated cable row	2 x 9–11	2 x 6–8
Diamond push-up (on knees if necessary)	2 x 10–15	2 x 15–20
One-arm standing twisting cable row	2 x 9–11	2 x 6–8
One-arm standing twisting cable chest press	2 x 9–11	2 x 6–8
Dumbbell bent-over lateral raise	2 x 9–11	2 x 6–8
Cable wood chop	2 x 9–11	2 x 6–8
Dumbbell hammer curl	2 x 9–11	2 x 6–8
Triceps rope push-down	2 x 9–11	2 x 6–8
Seated knee raise holding dumbbell between feet	2 x 9–11	2 x 6–8
Dumbbell side bend	2 x 20–25	2 x 15–20

Workout D (Lower body and core)		
Exercise	**Sets x Reps**	
	Weeks 1, 3, 5, 7, 9, 11	**Weeks 2, 4, 6, 8, 10, 12**
Barbell deadlift	2 x 9–11	2 x 6–8
Decline twisting sit-up	2 x 20–25	2 x 25–30
Dumbbell Bulgarian split squat	2 x 9–11	2 x 6–8
Single straight-leg dumbbell deadlift	2 x 9–11	2 x 6–8
Smith machine kneeling rear kick	2 x 9–11	2 x 6–8
Seated or lying leg curl	2 x 9–11	2 x 6–8
Machine seated calf raise	2 x 15–20	2 x 10–15
Hanging straight leg and hip raise	2 x 10–15	2 x 15–20
Cable hip abduction	2 x 9–11	2 x 6–8
Cable hip adduction	2 x 9–11	2 x 6–8

Alternatives for cable/machine exercises

- Medium-grip lat pull-down — Medium-grip band lat pull-down or medium-grip pull-up
- Cable face pull — Dumbbell face pull or band face pull
- Captain's chair leg and hip raise with dumbbell between feet — Hanging leg and hip raise with dumbbell between feet or lying leg and hip raise with bands attached to ankles
- Machine standing calf raise — Standing dumbbell one-leg calf raise or band standing calf raise
- Wheel rollout — Ab walkout or inch worm
- Hyperextension holding a plate against chest — Straight-leg deadlift
- Seated cable row — Bent-over dumbbell row, bent-over barbell row, or band row
- One-arm standing twisting cable row — One-arm standing twisting band row or dumbbell twisting row
- One-arm standing twisting cable chest press — One-arm standing twisting band chest press or one-arm dumbbell bench press
- Cable wood chop — Band wood chop, weighted lying oblique twist, or weighted Russian twist
- Triceps rope push-down — Barbell overhead triceps extension or band push-down
- Smith machine kneeling rear kick — Band rear kick or barbell one-leg glute bridge
- Seated or lying leg curl — Inverse leg curl, one-leg stability ball leg curl, or band leg curl
- Machine seated calf raise — Barbell seated calf raise
- Cable hip abduction — Band hip abduction or side plank hip abduction
- Cable hip adduction — Band hip adduction or side plank hip adduction

Women's Plateau Buster

Description

The 8-week Women's Plateau Buster is designed to:

- train all of your major muscle groups
- build muscle/curves in the 9–11 and 6–8 rep ranges
- strengthen your core and primal movement patterns
- introduce you to the pre-exhaustion intensity training protocol
- help you to break out of plateaus and keep making progress.

The program consists of three workouts (A, B, and C). Workout A will train your back, biceps, core, and inner and outer thighs; Workout B will train your chest, shoulders, triceps, and core; and Workout C will train your legs, glutes, and core.

In weeks 1, 3, 5, and 7, you will train in the 9–11 rep range; in weeks 2, 4, 6, and 8, you will train in the 6–8 rep range.

The exercises in each workout have been arranged in accordance with the pre-exhaustion protocol, which will ensure that your prime mover muscles are partially exhausted by isolation exercises before you move on to the major compound exercises. The pre-exhaustion is intended to boost muscular overload and amplify the stimulus for development, thus increasing the program's chances of helping you to "bust" through plateaus and never stop making progress. You can also use the program as an additional and advanced MCFS mesocycle ("MCFS 6").

Please read the **Overview of women's training programs**, at the beginning of this chapter, before you start this program.

Suitability

- Individuals who have completed Maximum Curves and Functional Strength 5
- Anyone who has at least 12 months of consistent weight training experience

Instructions

- Complete the workouts (A, B, and C) in the order presented.
- The recommend workout schedules are ABCX (i.e. three days on, one day off) or ABCXABX (i.e. three days on, one day off, two days on, one day off, and then continue the sequence from where you left off).
- Perform the exercises in the order presented.
- Rest for 30 to 90 seconds between sets.
- Rest for 1 to 2 minutes between exercises.
- Always use a weight that is heavy enough to make the reps challenging.

- Whenever you have to increase the weight, add a maximum of 5 lb (2.5 kg) to upper-body exercises or a maximum of 10 lb (5 kg) to lower-body exercises.
- Try to master the proper form of each exercise, including proper breathing technique. Instructions for most exercises are available on my website, **weighttraining.guide**. Also, try to develop a mental connection with your muscles and with the movement patterns.
- If you get bored of an exercise, see the **Overview of women's training programs** for alternatives.
- If training at home in the absence of cable machines and other specialized equipment, see below the exercise tables for exercise alternatives.
- Don't forget to warm up before, and cool down after, each workout.
- Once you have completed the Women's Plateau Buster, you must take a deload week. Only then can you repeat the program or one of the other programs.

Workout A (Back, biceps, core, inner and outer thighs)		
Exercise	**Sets x Reps**	
	Weeks 1, 3, 5, 7	**Weeks 2, 4, 6, 8**
Cable straight-arm pull-down	2 x 9–11	2 x 6–8
Pull-up	2 x 6–8	2 x 9–11
Seated cable row	2 x 9–11	2 x 6–8
Overhead cable curl	2 x 9–11	2 x 6–8
EZ bar curl	2 x 9–11	2 x 6–8
Wheel rollout	3 x 10–15	3 x 15–20
Hanging straight leg and hip raise	2 x 10–15	2 x 15–20
Cable hip abduction	2 x 9–11	2 x 6–8
Cable hip adduction	2 x 9–11	2 x 6–8

Workout B (Chest, shoulders, triceps, core)		
Exercise	**Sets x Reps**	
	Weeks 1, 3, 5, 7	**Weeks 2, 4, 6, 8**
Dumbbell fly	2 x 9–11	2 x 6–8
Push-up (on knees if necessary)	2 x 10–15	2 x 15–20
Alternating dumbbell front raise	2 x 9–11	2 x 6–8

1

Seated dumbbell overhead press	2 x 9–11	2 x 6–8
Dumbbell bent-over lateral raise	2 x 9–11	2 x 6–8
Cable face pull	2 x 9–11	2 x 6–8
Dumbbell kickback	2 x 9–11	2 x 6–8
Diamond push-up (on knees if necessary)	2 x 10–15	2 x 15–20
Bicycle crunch	3 x 20–25	3 x 25–30
Lying side hip raise	2 x 20–25	2 x 25–30

Workout C (Legs, glutes, core)		
Exercise	Sets x Reps	
	Weeks 1, 3, 5, 7	Weeks 2, 4, 6, 8
Barbell hip thrust	2 x 9–11	2 x 6–8
Dumbbell forward-leaning lunge	2 x 9–11	2 x 6–8
Barbell sumo squat	3 x 9–11	3 x 6–8
Seated or lying leg curl	2 x 9–11	2 x 6–8
Twisting hyperextension holding plate against chest	2 x 9–11	2 x 6–8
Barbell Romanian deadlift	2 x 9–11	2 x 6–8
Machine seated calf raise	2 x 15–20	2 x 10–15
Machine standing calf raise	3 x 15–20	3 x 10–15
Captain's chair leg and hip raise with dumbbell between feet	2 x 9–11	2 x 6–8

Alternatives for cable/machine exercises

- Cable straight-arm pull-down — Band straight-arm pull-down or dumbbell pull-over
- Seated cable row — Bent-over dumbbell row, bent-over barbell row, or band row
- Overhead cable curl — Concentration curl
- Wheel rollout — Ab walkout or inch worm
- Cable hip abduction — Band hip abduction or side plank hip abduction
- Cable hip adduction — Band hip adduction or side plank hip adduction
- Cable face pull — Dumbbell face pull or band face pull
- Seated or lying leg curl — Inverse leg curl, one-leg stability ball leg curl, or band leg curl

- Twisting hyperextension holding plate against chest — Twisting hyperextension on flat bench holding plate against chest
- Machine seated calf raise — Barbell seated calf raise
- Machine standing calf raise — Standing dumbbell one-leg calf raise or band standing calf raise
- Captain's chair leg and hip raise with dumbbell between feet — Hanging leg and hip raise with dumbbell between feet or lying leg and hip raise with bands attached to ankles

Minimalistic Program for Busy Women

Description

The 12-week Minimalistic Program for Busy Women is designed to:

- train all of your major muscle groups
- build muscle/curves in the 9–11 and 6–8 rep ranges
- strengthen your core and primal movement patterns
- introduce you to the intensity technique of superset training
- minimize the time it takes to get an effective full-body workout.

The program consists of two workouts (A and B). Workout A will train your upper body and core; Workout B will train your lower body and core.

The exercises in all of the workouts have been arranged into supersets, which makes the workouts short and intense.

In weeks 1, 3, 5, 7, 9, and 11, you will train in the 9–11 rep range; in weeks 2, 4, 6, 8, 10, and 12, you will train in the 6–8 rep range.

Please read the **Overview of women's training programs**, at the beginning of this chapter, before you start this program.

Suitability

- Individuals who have completed at least microcycles 1–3 of the Women's Beginner program
- Anyone who has at least 3 months of consistent weight training experience

Instructions

- Complete each workout (A and B) twice per week, in the order presented.
- The recommend workout schedule is ABXABXX (where "X" is a rest day). Try not to train four days on and three days off (i.e. ABABXXX).

- The exercises are arranged into pairs as supersets. After you complete one set of the first exercise, perform a set of the second exercise without resting.
- Rest for 1 to 2 minutes before repeating the superset and before moving on to the next superset.
- Always use a weight that is heavy enough to make the reps challenging.
- Whenever you have to increase the weight, add a maximum of 5 lb (2.5 kg) to upper-body exercises or a maximum of 10 lb (5 kg) to lower-body exercises.
- Try to master the proper form of each exercise, including proper breathing technique. Instructions for most exercises are available on my website, **weighttraining.guide**. Also, try to develop a mental connection with your muscles and with the movement patterns.
- If you get bored of an exercise, see the **Overview of women's training programs** for alternatives.
- If training at home in the absence of cable machines and other specialized equipment, see below the exercise tables for exercise alternatives.
- Don't forget to warm up before, and cool down after, each workout.
- Once you have completed the Minimalistic Program for Busy Women, you must take a deload week. Only then can you repeat the program or start the MCFS programs.

Workout A (Upper body and core)		
Exercise	**Sets x Reps**	
	Weeks 1, 3, 5, 7, 9, 11	**Weeks 2, 4, 6, 8, 10, 12**
Seated cable row	2 x 9–11	2 x 6–8
Push-up (on knees if necessary)	2 x 10–15	2 x 15–20
Medium-grip lat pull-down	2 x 9–11	2 x 6–8
Seated dumbbell overhead press	2 x 9–11	2 x 6–8
Cable face pull	2 x 9–11	2 x 6–8
Weighted bench dip	2 x 9–11	2 x 6–8
Dumbbell curl	2 x 9–11	2 x 6–8
Wheel rollout	2 x 10–15	2 x 15–20

Workout B (Lower body and core)		
Exercise	**Sets x Reps**	
	Weeks 1, 3, 5, 7, 9, 11	**Weeks 2, 4, 6, 8, 10, 12**
Barbell sumo squat	2 x 9–11	2 x 6–8
Dumbbell Romanian deadlift	2 x 9–11	2 x 6–8
Dumbbell forward-leaning lunge	2 x 9–11	2 x 6–8

Seated or lying leg curl	2 x 9–11	2 x 6–8
Captain's chair leg and hip raise	2 x 10–15	2 x 15–20
Machine standing calf raise	2 x 15–20	2 x 10–15
Bicycle crunch	2 x 25–30	2 x 30–35

Alternatives for cable/machine exercises

- Seated cable row — Bent-over dumbbell row, bent-over barbell row, or band row
- Medium-grip lat pull-down — Medium-grip band lat pull-down or medium-grip self-assisted pull-up
- Cable face pull — Dumbbell face pull or band face pull
- Wheel rollout — Ab walkout or inch worm
- Seated or lying leg curl — Inverse leg curl, one-leg stability ball leg curl, or band leg curl
- Captain's chair leg and hip raise — Lying or hanging leg and hip raise
- Machine standing calf raise — Standing dumbbell one-leg calf raise or band standing calf raise

PART 4: BODYWEIGHT, POWER, AND PLYOMETRIC WORKOUTS

Chapter 9: Bodyweight training

Fundamentals of bodyweight training

What is bodyweight training?

Bodyweight training involves performing exercises that use your own body weight as resistance. Some of the exercises require basic equipment, such as a pull-up bar or stability ball, whereas other exercises require no equipment. The wheel rollout, inverted shrug, and stability ball pike are examples of exercises that require basic equipment, whereas the one-arm push-up, reverse plank, and handstand press are examples of exercises that do not require equipment.

What are the benefits of bodyweight training?

Bodyweight training can help you to:

- master your own body weight
- develop functional strength
- improve your agility, coordination, and balance
- build an impressive baseline of muscular size and strength
- significantly increase your muscular endurance
- burn calories
- lose weight
- enhance your overall fitness and athleticism.

You can also perform bodyweight training almost anywhere (for example, at home, at the park, and on vacation), and you obviously don't have to pay any gym fees.

How effective is bodyweight training?

If your goal includes any of the benefits listed above, then bodyweight training can be very effective and useful. However, if your goal is to build extensive muscle or curves or develop significant strength, then bodyweight training will not take you very far. The reason is that, as made clear in the **Weight Training Guide**, in **How many sets and reps should I do?**, in order to build muscle/curves or strength, you have to train with heavy weights, and you have to keep increasing the amount of weight that you use. With bodyweight training, the amount of resistance that you have to work with is obviously limited by your body weight, thus limiting your potential to build muscle and strength. Simply increasing the number of reps that you complete will not work because this will mainly lead to the development of muscular endurance, not muscular size and strength.

There are some measures that you can take to increase the level of resistance, such as wear a weighted vest or rucksack, or wrap a chain around your torso. However, strictly speaking, these exercises will no longer be bodyweight exercises. Other measures that you can take to increase resistance or tension without the use of auxiliary items do exist, but their effects are still limited. Such measures include:

- changing the movement pattern of the exercise (for example, performing the archer pull-up instead of the standard pull-up)
- adjusting the leverage used in the exercise (for example, performing the wheel rollout while standing instead of while kneeling)
- using one limb instead of two (for example, performing the pistol squat instead of the bodyweight squat)
- adding isometric pauses or "pulses" to the exercise (for example, pausing for a few seconds at the top of a reverse crunch, or pulsing a few times at the bottom of a bodyweight squat)
- adding explosiveness to the movements (such as performing squat jumps instead of bodyweight squats)
- slowing the exercise down so as to increase the muscles' time under tension.

I should also mention that just as bodyweight exercises can be progressed to increase resistance or tension, they can also be regressed to suit a lower level of fitness or strength. This makes bodyweight training suitable for a wide range of fitness levels. For example, the push-up can be performed on the knees, and the leg raise can be performed while lying down instead of while hanging.

Another limitation of bodyweight training is that balancing the training programs is relatively difficult. There are many more pushing exercises than there are pulling exercises, and the pulling exercises often require basic equipment (such as a pull-up bar), whereas the pushing exercises often do not.

Equipment-free bodyweight workouts

Below I present two full-body bodyweight workouts, one for men and one for women. The workouts require no equipment apart from items of furniture. You can use the workouts if you can't make it to the gym and lack home equipment. You can also use them to help preserve your physique or figure when you go on short vacations.

In addition to the workouts, I have provided a table of bodyweight exercises (Table 9.1), along with instructions on how to design your own mainly-equipment-free bodyweight workouts. As you'll notice, I've made the process as easy as possible for you. Being able to design your own bodyweight workouts will allow you to incorporate lots of variation into your training, which will keep you engaged and your body challenged.

Please use my website, **weighttraining.guide**, to learn how to perform the exercises in proper form. If you can't find an exercise on my website, please check YouTube. Explaining the proper form of every exercise is beyond the scope of this chapter.

Workout instructions

- Complete the workout either every other day (AX) or three days a week (AXAXAXX).
- Rest for only 20 to 30 seconds between sets.

- Rest for only 60 to 90 seconds between exercises.
- Try to increase the number of reps that you perform.
- Warm up before the workout with five minutes of dynamic stretching.
- Cool down after the workout with five minutes of static stretching.

Body parts	Exercise	Sets x Reps
Glutes, quadriceps	Bulgarian split squat	3 x 12–14
Hamstrings	Inverse leg curl (Lock your feet under your sofa)	2 x 15–20
Calves	Standing single-leg calf raise (Stand on the edge of a step)	3 x 25–30
Back, posterior shoulders, biceps	Inverted row (You can do this lying under a chair)	3 x 12–14
Chest, anterior shoulders, triceps	Chest dip (Suspend your body between two sturdy surfaces)	3 x 12–14
Lower back	Superman	2 x 25–30
Abs, hip flexors, obliques	Bicycle crunch	2 x 25–30

Equipment-free bodyweight workout for men.

Body parts	Exercise	Sets x Reps
Glutes, quadriceps	Step-up	3 x 12–14
Glutes	Single-leg hip thrust	2 x 15–20
Hamstrings	Single straight-leg deadlift	2 x 15–20
Calves	Standing single-leg calf raise (Stand on the edge of a step)	2 x 25–30
Back, posterior shoulders, biceps	Inverted row (You can do this lying under a chair)	2 x 12–14
Chest, anterior shoulders, triceps	Push-up (on knees if necessary)	2 x 12–14
Lower back	Superman	2 x 25–30
Abs, hip flexors, obliques	Bicycle crunch	3 x 25–30

Equipment-free bodyweight workout for women.

How to design your own equipment-free bodyweight workouts

Instructions

Refer to Table 9.1. Choose at least one exercise from each of the following rows:

- Quadriceps, glutes
- Hamstrings
- Calves
- Back, posterior shoulders, biceps
- Chest, anterior shoulders, triceps
- Lower back
- Abs, hip flexors
- Obliques

Any other exercises that you choose will be a bonus. Men might want to choose additional exercises for biceps and triceps, whereas women might want to choose additional exercises for glutes and inner/outer thighs.

Arrange the exercises in the same order as the rows are presented in Table 9.1 (for example, back exercises should come before biceps exercises).

Perform at least two sets of each exercise, following the same instructions as I presented for the bodyweight workouts that I designed.

Body part	Exercises
Quadriceps, glutes	Bodyweight squat, Squat jump, Split squat, Bulgarian split squat, Pistol squat, Step-up, Lunge, Jumping lunge
Quadriceps	Sissy squat
Glutes	Single-leg glute bridge, Single-leg hip thrust
Hamstrings	Inverse leg curl, Single straight-leg deadlift, Lying single straight-leg hip extension
Inner thighs	Side plank hip adduction
Outer thighs	Side plank hip abduction
Calves	Standing single-leg calf raise
Back, posterior shoulders, biceps	Pull-up, Chin-up, Inverted row, One-arm towel row

Back, posterior shoulders	Elbow lift/Reverse push-up
Chest, anterior shoulders, triceps	Chest dip, Push-up, Decline push-up, Pike push-up
Anterior and lateral shoulders, triceps	Pike press, Handstand press (Can be dangerous!)
Triceps	Diamond push-up, Triceps dip, Bench dip, Bodyweight triceps extension
Biceps	Biceps leg curl, Side-lying biceps bodyweight curl
Lower back	Superman, Alternating superman, Bird dog, Reverse plank
Abs, Hip flexors	Bicycle crunch, Lying leg and hip raise, Sit-up, Jack-knife sit-up, V-up, Seated leg raise, Front plank
Abs	Reverse crunch, Vertical leg crunch
Hip flexors	Lying leg raise, Scissor kick
Obliques	Bicycle crunch, Russian twist, Lying oblique twist, Lying side hip raise, Lying heel touch, Side crunch, Side plank

Table 9.1. Bodyweight exercises that you can use to put together your own mainly-equipment-free bodyweight workouts.

Chapter 10: Power and plyometric training

Fundamentals of power and plyometric training

What is muscular power?

Muscular power is different from muscular strength. Muscular strength is the amount of force that your muscle can produce, whereas muscular power is the amount of strength and speed that your muscle can produce.

How is muscular power developed?

Muscular power is developed by performing exercises that involve rapidly generating a large amount of force. Exercises for the lower body often involve hopping and jumping (for example, the broad jump and box jump). Exercises for the upper body usually involve barbell weightlifting movements (for example, the snatch), as well as advanced push-up variations (for example, the clap push-up), and rapid medicine ball catching and throwing actions (for example, the chest throw).

What is plyometric training?

You will often hear the word "plyometric" being used to describe power training, especially jump training. However, true plyometric training is a little different. It is an advanced type of power training specifically designed to harness the muscles' and tendons' ability to store and then rapidly release energy.

The most popular plyometric exercise is probably the platform depth jump. It involves stepping off a low platform or box, dropping vertically, absorbing the landing by flexing the hips and knees, and then immediately launching into a jump, usually onto a high box or over a hurdle. During the landing after the initial drop, the muscles are forced to eccentrically contract and stretch in order to prevent the body from collapsing. The tendons, which attach the muscles to bones, stretch even more than do the muscles. Most of the gravitational energy that enters the muscles and tendons is lost as heat, while some of it is temporarily stored. In order to launch into an immediate jump, the muscles then concentrically contract. The force of the concentric contraction coupled with the energy that was stored within the muscles and tendons produces a more explosive movement than would have occurred if the initial eccentric contraction had not taken place.

Because the muscles and tendons stretch during the eccentric contraction and shorten during the concentric contraction, the whole process is known as the **stretch-shortening cycle (SSC)**. The transition between the eccentric and concentric contractions is known as the **amortization phase**. In order for an exercise to be considered truly plyometric, the amortization phase must be extremely short, ideally taking no longer than 0.25 seconds. The reason is that in exercises in which the amortization phase takes longer, the stored energy is dissipated as heat and the plyometric effect is lost. Although such exercises can be used to develop power and to prepare for plyometric exercises, they should not themselves be deemed plyometric.

What are the benefits of power and plyometric training?

Power and plyometric training can help you to:

- develop explosive power
- increase the height and length of your jump
- boost your running speed
- improve your coordination, balance, and agility
- enhance your reflexes and reaction times
- develop functional strength
- strengthen your muscles, bones, tendons, and ligaments
- reduce your risk of sporting injuries
- improve your athleticism and sporting performance.

Power and plyometric workouts

Below I present two power workouts and one plyometric workout that you can occasionally use in place of a weight training or cardio workout. The workouts are not suitable for beginners because the explosive nature of the exercises makes them risky. Therefore, before trying a workout, please refer to its suitability criteria.

An important point to keep in mind regarding power and especially plyometric training is that the focus should always be on quality rather than quantity. You are trying to develop a skill more than you are trying to condition your muscles, tendons, and central nervous system. Therefore, take your time with the exercises and try to focus. This is also important for your safety.

Please use YouTube and other resources to learn how to perform the exercises in good form. Explaining the proper form of the exercises is beyond the scope of this chapter.

Make sure that you are fully warmed up before you start a power or plyometric workout. Five minutes of dynamic stretching followed by five minutes of jogging should suffice. You should also cool down after each workout with five minutes of static stretching.

Power workout 1: Lower body

- Power workout 1 is designed to help you to develop lower-body power and agility, as well as improve your jumping and sprinting abilities
- Suitability: Anyone who has completed the beginner weight training program
- Equipment required: Box
- Rest for 2 to 5 minutes between sets and exercises
- As you gain experience, try to gradually increase how high or far you jump, or how fast you move

Exercise	Sets x Reps
Front box jump	3 x 5
Broad jump	3 x 5
Skater jump	3 x 30–45 s
Box lateral shuffle	3 x 30–45 s
s = seconds	

Power workout 2: Upper body

- Power workout 2 is designed to help you to develop the power of your upper body and core
- Suitability: Anyone who has more than 6 months of weight training experience
- Equipment required: Barbell
- Rest for 2 to 5 minutes between sets and exercises
- If new to the exercises, start off very lightly and learn proper form. Once you gather experience, start adding weight until the reps become challenging

Exercise	Sets x Reps
Clean	3 x 3–5
Snatch	3 x 3–5
Clean and jerk	3 x 3–5
Clap push-up (on knees if necessary)	3 x 5–10

Plyometric workout

- The plyometric workout is designed to help you to improve the explosive performance of your upper body, lower body, and core
- Suitability: Anyone who has more than 6 months of weight training experience and who has mastered the power workouts
- Equipment required: Boxes, a medicine ball, and a wall against which to throw the ball
- Rest for 2 to 5 minutes between sets and exercises
- For the two depth jump exercises, make sure that the platform or box from which you drop isn't too tall. The reason is that the taller the box is, the longer your amortization phase will be. Your goal while performing the depth jump exercises is to increase the height or distance of your jump while keeping the amortization phase below 0.25 seconds

- For the two throwing exercises, choose a medicine ball of a suitable weight. Your goal during these exercises is to catch and launch the ball back at the wall as quickly as possible. As you get stronger and faster, increase the weight of the ball

Exercise	Sets x Reps
Platform depth jump	3 x 3–5
Long depth jump	3 x 3–5
Chest throw (against a wall)	3 x 30–45 s
Seated or standing side throw (against a wall)	4 x 30–45 s
s = seconds	

PART 5: CARDIO GUIDE

Chapter 11: Cardiovascular training

Introduction to the Cardio Guide

Cardiovascular training (cardio) is very important for overall health and fitness. No well-rounded physical fitness program is complete without both weight training and cardio. Although many of the fitness benefits of the two types of training do overlap, there are some benefits that can only be derived to a significant degree from cardio (such as improved cardiovascular fitness and endurance) and some benefits that can only be derived to a significant degree from weight training (such as increased muscular size and strength). Stretching and functional training are also important for complete fitness; however, these can be incorporated into the weight training and cardio training programs (as I have in this book).

The purpose of the Cardio Guide, which consists of two chapters, is to provide you with everything you need in order to safely and successfully improve your cardiovascular fitness and endurance using effective cardiovascular training. I begin the first chapter with a very brief overview of the basics of exercise physiology, an understanding of which will be necessary to fully grasp the concepts that arise in this and the second chapter. I then explain what cardio is, why it's beneficial, how to calculate your training zones, and how to use cardio effectively. The first chapter concludes with an exploration of the applications, advantages, and disadvantages of the three main types of cardio: steady-state training, interval training, and circuit training.

In the second chapter, I provide three cardio training programs with interchangeable workouts. There's a steady-state program with three workouts, an interval training program with three workouts, and a functional circuit training program with two workouts. The workouts cater for all levels of experience, from beginner to advanced, and can be progressed as your fitness improves. The second chapter concludes with an explanation of how to design your own functional circuit training cardio workouts.

Important!

If you've been living an inactive lifestyle, cardio of a vigorous intensity may be a little risky for you. The risk is increased by old age, obesity, diabetes, abnormal cholesterol levels, high blood pressure, smoking, and drinking, as well as having a family history of coronary heart disease. If any of these apply to you, please seek medical clearance before trying cardio or starting any training program.

Basics of exercise physiology

Your two energy systems

Your muscle cells need **energy** to survive and work. When you eat food, the food is broken down into **nutrients**, such as fat, protein, and carbohydrate, by your **digestive system**. The nutrients are pumped around your body, to your muscle cells, by your **cardiovascular system** (heart and blood vessels). Your muscle cells take the nutrients in and break them down to release energy, which they store in special molecules called **adenosine triphosphate (ATP)**. Your muscle cells can then use the energy stored inside the ATP molecules to fuel their work.

The process of making ATP is known as **cellular respiration**. Cellular respiration can occur either with oxygen or without oxygen. The chemical pathway that utilizes oxygen to make ATP is known as **aerobic respiration**, whereas the chemical pathway that doesn't utilize oxygen is known as **anaerobic respiration**. The oxygen is drawn into your body from the air by your **respiratory system** (lungs, diaphragm, and breathing muscles) and pumped around your body by your cardiovascular system.

Aerobic respiration burns fat and carbohydrate (and protein only when fat and carbohydrate are low), and produces lots of ATP via a long, four-stage process (Table 13.1). The stages occur within the **cytoplasm** (inner fluid) and **mitochondria** (energy-producing organelles) of the cells. In contrast, anaerobic respiration mainly burns carbohydrate (and protein when carbohydrate is low) and produces comparatively very little ATP via a short, two-stage process. The stages take place only within the cytoplasm. As such, compared with aerobic respiration, anaerobic respiration is much faster but far less efficient at producing ATP.

	Aerobic respiration	Anaerobic respiration
Oxygen required?	Yes	No
Reactants	Fat and carbohydrate; protein if fat and carbohydrate are low	Carbohydrate; protein if carbohydrate is low
Stages	Glycolysis Link reaction Krebs Cycle Electron Transport Chain	Glycolysis Fermentation
Locations	Cytoplasm and mitochondria	Cytoplasm
Energy (ATP) yield	30–38	2

Table 13.1. A comparison of aerobic and anaerobic respiration, including oxygen requirement, reactants, number of stages, locations of occurrence, and energy yields.

What happens when you exercise?

When you exercise, both aerobic respiration and anaerobic respiration occur within your muscle cells at the same time. However, the energy system that is relied upon the most at any moment in time depends on how rapidly your cells need to make ATP.

When you first start to exercise, your cells use anaerobic respiration to derive a rapid supply of energy. If the exercise continues for over a minute or so and is of a light to moderate intensity, aerobic respiration starts to kick in and take over. The main source of fuel at this point for aerobic respiration is **fat**. However, if the intensity of the exercise increases, aerobic respiration starts to burn an increasing amount of **carbohydrate** instead. What's more, to keep up with the demand for oxygen and nutrients, the cardiovascular and respiratory systems (together known as the **cardiorespiratory system**) speed up.

If the intensity of the exercise continues to increase, at a certain point of intensity, the cells start to require a more rapid source of energy than aerobic respiration can provide. Therefore, anaerobic respiration starts to play a more significant role.

In order to rapidly produce ATP, anaerobic respiration mainly burns stores of carbohydrate in your muscle cells known as **glycogen**. The process of breaking down glycogen to make ATP produces **lactate** and releases **hydrogen ions** into your muscles, which your body can process up to a certain point of intensity. However, if the intensity of the exercise becomes vigorous and anaerobic respiration really takes off, lactate and hydrogen ions start to accumulate in the muscles. The ions (not the lactate) lower the muscles' pH level in a process known as **metabolic acidosis**, which you experience as **fatigue**. After a while, the fatigue forces you to stop the exercise so that the cells can clear themselves and the system can be restored. The duration for which you can tolerate vigorous exercise is known as your level of **endurance**.

What factors limit your endurance?

The point of intensity at which hydrogen ions and lactate are produced faster than they can be processed is known as your **lactate threshold**. Your lactate threshold is a good indicator of your level of endurance. You generally reach your lactate threshold when your heartbeat increases to between 80% and 90% of its maximum rate.

Your level of endurance is also affected by your body's ability to take in and utilize oxygen. The maximum amount of oxygen that your body can utilize during exercise is known as your **VO_2 max** (maximum volume of oxygen) or **aerobic capacity**. Generally speaking, the more oxygen you can utilize, the better, faster, and longer you can perform. VO_2 max is affected by a number of factors, including the efficiency of your cardiorespiratory system and the availability of fat-burning enzymes and mitochondria (the organelles in which aerobic respiration takes place) in your muscle cells.

Your VO_2 max rests above your lactate threshold. In other words, the accumulation of lactate and hydrogen ions occurs before your body even starts to utilize oxygen to its full potential. As such, you can think of your VO_2 max as being your aerobic endurance potential, whereas you can think of your lactate threshold as being a factor that can limit your ability to tap that potential.

The great news is that by using **cardiovascular training**, you should be able to increase your VO_2 max and especially your lactate threshold, thus dramatically improving your level of endurance and other performance-related abilities.

Fundamentals of cardiovascular training

What is cardiovascular training?

Cardiovascular training is any physical exercise or activity that is used to improve endurance and cardiorespiratory fitness. Since it burns a lot of calories, cardio is also often used for the process of losing weight.

In its most basic form (known as **steady-state training**), cardio involves performing an exercise (such as jogging or cycling) at a prescribed **intensity** for a prescribed period of time. As you will soon learn, training at different intensities for different durations helps to develop different aspects of health and cardiorespiratory fitness.

What are the benefits of cardio?

Depending on how you train, cardio can:

- improve the strength and efficiency of your cardiorespiratory system
- increase your VO$_2$ max and lactate threshold
- boost your aerobic and anaerobic metabolisms
- increase your energy levels
- reduce your blood pressure and resting heart rate
- strengthen your bones, tendons, and ligaments
- increase your high-density lipoprotein (i.e. "good" cholesterol) and reduce your overall cholesterol
- reduce your risks of heart disease, stroke, osteoporosis, and certain types of cancer
- increase your insulin sensitivity, which reduces your risk of developing diabetes
- boost your immune system
- enhance your mental health and cognitive capabilities
- dramatically improve your endurance and overall level of fitness.

In the context of weight training, cardio can help in the process of muscular repair and development by speeding up the delivery of oxygen and nutrients to, and the removal of waste products from, your muscles. Muscle growth is also aided by the increase in insulin sensitivity, which helps your muscle cells to better absorb nutrients.

What are the official recommendations for cardio?

For cardiorespiratory health and fitness, the American College of Sports Medicine (ACSM) recommends any one of the following:

- 30 to 60 minutes of moderate-intensity exercise for 5 days a week
- 20 to 60 minutes of vigorous-intensity exercise for 3 days a week
- A combination of both moderate- and vigorous-intensity exercise for 3 to 5 days a week

Beginners who have been sedentary (very inactive) for several months should start with light-intensity exercise and gradually build up to meet the above recommendations.

How do you measure exercise intensity?

The ACSM defines five levels of exercise intensity, as presented in Table 13.2. Each level is defined based on a range of **maximum heart rate (HR_{max})**. For example, moderate-intensity exercise is defined as exercise that forces your heart to beat at between 64% and 76% of its maximum rate, whereas vigorous-intensity exercise is defined as exercise that forces your heart to beat at between 77% and 95% of its maximum rate.

Intensity	% HR_{max}	% $HR_{reserve}$	RPE	Training effects and notes
Very light (Aerobic)	<57	<30	6–8	Basic health Minor improvements in fitness Not considered exercise
Light (Aerobic)	57–63	30–39	9–11	Basic fitness Suitable for warming up and cooling down
Moderate (Aerobic)	64–76	40–59	12–13	Cardiorespiratory fitness Aerobic capacity and endurance Burn more fat than carbohydrate
Vigorous (Anaerobic after ~85% HR_{max})	77–95	60–89	14–17	Advanced cardiorespiratory fitness Advanced aerobic capacity and endurance Burn more carbohydrate than fat *From ~85% HR_{max} (lactate threshold):* Anaerobic capacity Lactate tolerance Type II muscle fiber recruitment Speed, power, and performance Mostly burn glycogen stored in muscles Increased risk of injury
Near-maximal to maximal (Anaerobic)	≥96	≥90	18–20	Advanced anaerobic capacity Advanced lactate tolerance Maximal Type II muscle fiber recruitment Maximum speed, power, and performance Advanced individuals only Short bursts only Highest potential for injury

Table 13.2. Exercise intensity levels as defined by the ACSM, including the range of maximum heart rate (HR_{max}), range of reserve heart rate ($HR_{reserve}$), rating of perceived exertion (RPE), and training effects and notes associated with each level. The training effects and notes were added by me.

Each level of intensity can also be defined based on a range of **heart rate reserve (HR$_{reserve}$)** instead of HR$_{max}$. HR$_{reserve}$ is the difference between your HR$_{max}$ and your **resting heart rate (HR$_{resting}$)**. In other words, HR$_{reserve}$ is what's left after you subtract your HR$_{resting}$ from your HR$_{max}$. Since fitter individuals have a lower HR$_{resting}$, calculating exercise intensity based on HR$_{reserve}$ is more accurate than calculating it based on HR$_{max}$ because the HR$_{reserve}$ calculation takes the personal level of fitness into account.

As you can see from Table 13.2, each level of intensity is also associated with a **rating of perceived exertion (RPE)**. This is a numerical rating that you can use to subjectively estimate your level of exercise intensity if you don't know how to calculate intensity based on HR$_{max}$ or HR$_{reserve}$. The RPE scale ranges from 6 to 20 because it is designed to also help you to estimate your heart rate. All you have to do is multiply the rate by 10 to get a very rough estimate. The RPE scale is also useful if you suffer from an abnormal heart rate or take heart-rate-affecting medications (such as beta-blockers), which make your heart rate an unreliable indication of exercise intensity.

You can view each level of intensity in Table 13.2 as a **training zone**. Training in different zones leads to different **training effects**. The training effects associated with each training zone were added by me; they were not defined by the ACSM. The training effects that I added give you a general idea of the kinds of effects that you could expect to observe if you were to start cardiovascular training as a sedentary beginner and gradually progress through the different levels of intensity.

Note that there is no "Fat-Burning Zone", which is a widely held myth in cardiovascular training. As mentioned above, in the **Basics of exercise physiology**, your body will burn a higher percentage of fat than carbohydrate at lower intensities of training; however, at higher intensities, it will burn more total calories, which makes training at higher intensities better for weight loss.

How do you calculate your training zones?

As explained above, you can calculate your training zones in two different ways:

1. Using your HR$_{max}$
2. Using your HR$_{reserve}$

The first method is the easiest and is adequate for most gym-goers who are interested in general fitness. However, it is not as accurate as the second method, which also takes your personal level of fitness into account.

Note that your HR$_{max}$ doesn't change as you get fitter, whereas your HR$_{resting}$ does change. Therefore, if you use HR$_{reserve}$ to calculate your training zones, you will have to recalculate your training zones every couple of months.

Using HR$_{max}$

Your HR$_{max}$ is the highest number of times your heart can beat per minute during extremely intense (all-out) exercise. It usually decreases as you get older by about one beat per minute, starting from between the ages of 10 to 15.

The best way to get an accurate measure of your HR$_{max}$ is to undertake a **cardiac stress test** in a hospital or clinical setting, which, of course, isn't practical for everyone. Most people therefore estimate their HR$_{max}$ using the **Fox and Haskell equation** (HR$_{max}$ = 220 − age in years). However, this method has no scientific basis and has a large margin of error. A more accurate method — albeit one that still has a small margin of error — is to use the **Inbar equation**:

HR$_{max}$ = 205.8 − (0.685 × age)

For example, if you're 25 years old, your equation would look like this:

0.685 x 25 = 17.1

HR$_{max}$ = 205.8 − 17.1 = 189 beats per minute (bpm)

Once you know your HR$_{max}$, you can calculate your personal training zones by multiplying your HR$_{max}$ by the decimal equivalents of the zone ranges. For example, if you want to train within the moderate-intensity zone (64% to 76% of HR$_{max}$), your calculations would look like this:

64% of HR$_{max}$ = 189 x 0.64 = 121 bpm

76% of HR$_{max}$ = 189 x 0.76 = 144 bpm

Using HR$_{reserve}$

In order to use your HR$_{reserve}$ to calculate your training zones, in addition to your HR$_{max}$, you will need your HR$_{resting}$. To measure your HR$_{resting}$, just take your pulse in the mornings before you get out of bed, a couple of minutes after your alarm clock sounds. Do this for three days in a row and use the average.

To take your pulse, simply place your index finger and middle finger on your wrist, under the base of your thumb, where you will find your **radial pulse**. Count how many beats you feel for 15 seconds, and multiply it by four to get your beats per minute.

You can also take your pulse on your neck. Gently press the same two fingers on the side of your neck, in the hollow area just beside your wind pipe, where you will find your **carotid pulse**.

Once you have your HR$_{max}$ and HR$_{resting}$, plug them into the following equation, known as the **Karvonen formula**:

Target heart rate = ((HR$_{max}$ – HR$_{resting}$) x Intensity) + HR$_{resting}$

Notice that after you get your HR$_{reserve}$ by subtracting your HR$_{resting}$ from your HR$_{max}$, you multiply your HR$_{reserve}$ by the desired level of intensity, before adding your HR$_{resting}$ back on. As such, the level of intensity is only applied to HR$_{reserve}$. Here's an example calculation.

If your HR$_{max}$ is 189, your HR$_{resting}$ is 65, and you want to train in the vigorous-intensity zone (60% to 89% of HR$_{reserve}$), your equation would look like this:

HR$_{reserve}$ = 189 – 65 = 124 bpm

60% of HR$_{reserve}$ = (124 x 0.60 = 74) + 65 = 139 bpm

89% of HR$_{reserve}$ = (124 x 0.89 = 110) + 65 = 175 bpm

How do you monitor your heart rate during exercise?

Many of the machines that you can use for cardio have sensors built into their handles that can track your heart rate. However, the best way to monitor your heart rate is to use a fitness band. If you don't have one, you can take your heart rate manually via your radial or carotid pulses. Simply stop the exercise momentarily, take your pulse for six seconds, and multiply it by 10. This will give you your beats per minute.

In addition to monitoring your heart rate during exercise, you should always consider your **perceived effort**. The reason is that your heart rate can vary from day to day due to several factors, including diet, temperature, stress, emotions, and level of hydration. Taking into account both your heart rate and perceived exertion will give you a better idea of your performance and progress.

Types of cardio

So far, I have only covered the most basic form of cardio, known as **steady-state training**. However, there are two other popular types of cardio:

1. Interval training
2. Circuit training

The three types of cardio are quite different and offer different benefits. Let's look at the applications, advantages, and disadvantages of each type separately, as well as the exercises and activities that are most suitable for each type. You can then use the different types of cardio in a strategic fashion, in accordance with your goals, preferences, and level of experience.

Steady-state training

What is steady-state training?

As you are aware, steady-state training (SST) involves increasing your heart rate to a target training zone and keeping it there for a prescribed period of time. The benefits that you derive depend on the zone in which you choose to train.

Applications of SST

Although advanced individuals can use SST in the anaerobic zones to develop anaerobic metabolism, it is usually confined to the aerobic zones and used to develop aerobic metabolism and endurance.

Improving aerobic metabolism is extremely important because the majority of the physical functions and activities that your body undertakes (for example, digestion, breathing, walking, and sleeping) are powered by the aerobic metabolism. Even anaerobic exercises, such as sprinting, rely on the aerobic metabolism to restore the body to neutral after exercise. That's why anaerobic exercises force you to breathe heavily even though they themselves require little oxygen. Since all physical functions and activities rely on your aerobic metabolism, having a weak aerobic "engine" will limit everything you can do. By strengthening your aerobic metabolism using SST, you will be able to perform better at everything else.

Advantages of SST

- Great for developing VO_2 max, aerobic metabolism, and endurance
- Improves VO_2 max and aerobic metabolism by boosting the efficiency of your cardiorespiratory system and increasing the density of mitochondria and fat-burning enzymes in your muscle cells
- By enhancing your aerobic metabolism, reduces your body's demand for anaerobic respiration at more vigorous levels of intensity. This delays the onset of your lactate threshold, which enables you to train at a higher percentage of your VO_2 max
- Decreases your blood pressure and heart rate, both at rest and during exercise, as a result of improving cardiorespiratory efficiency. In turn, the reduced blood pressure and heart rate enhance your ability to relax and focus
- By increasing the availability of fat-burning enzymes in your muscle cells, enhances your body's ability to use fat as a fuel source
- Not as stressful on the cardiorespiratory system as is interval training
- Generates less metabolic waste and cellular damage than interval training
- Workouts can be recovered from relatively quickly

Disadvantages of SST

- Doesn't build strength, power, or muscle mass beyond a very low baseline level
- The lengthy workouts can be very boring for some people (Tip: Try listening to an audiobook)
- Its repetitive nature can increase the risk of repetitive stress injuries
- If used excessively, can lead to muscle loss, especially in the presence of inadequate caloric intake and in the absence of weight training

Suitable exercises for SST

Exercises and activities that are most suitable for SST include:

- Aerobics
- Dancing
- Swimming
- Jogging and running
- Stair climbing
- Cycling
- Rowing
- Elliptical cross-training

All of these activities allow you to increase and maintain a heart rate sufficient for aerobic training. With some activities, you increase your heart rate by increasing your pace (for example, jogging and swimming); with other activities, you can increase your heart rate by either increasing your pace or the level of resistance (for example, the rowing machine).

The best exercises and activities for SST are those that get the major muscles of both your upper body and lower body involved, while keeping the stress and impact on your joints to a minimum. Of course, it's best to alternate the types of exercises and activities that you use so as to avoid getting bored, as well as prevent your body from adapting, becoming more efficient at the exercise or activity, and using less energy.

Interval training

What is interval training?

Interval training involves alternating between different training zones in the same workout, for example, repeatedly switching between five-minute intervals of moderate-intensity and vigorous-intensity exercise. This kind of training can significantly increase the total volume and/or average exercise intensity that you perform. An advanced and very popular form of interval training, known as **high-intensity interval training (HIIT)**, involves alternating between very brief intervals of maximal-intensity exercise and longer intervals of moderate-intensity recovery exercise.

Applications of interval training

Interval training, especially HIIT, is usually used to improve anaerobic metabolism and lactate tolerance. However, since it involves alternating between intervals of lower and higher intensity exercise, it of course also improves aerobic metabolism.

Advantages of interval training

- Improves anaerobic metabolism by increasing the amount of enzymes that are necessary for anaerobic respiration
- By boosting anaerobic metabolism, empowers you to work at higher intensities for longer and with much more efficiency

- Improves your body's ability to transition between aerobic and anaerobic metabolisms (known as your **metabolic flexibility**)
- Enhances your lactate tolerance
- Improves explosive sporting performance
- More effective than SST at strengthening your cardiorespiratory system because it gets your heart, lungs, and breathing apparatus working much more vigorously
- The workouts are shorter and can therefore be less boring
- The intensity of the workouts, especially HIIT workouts, activates Type II muscle fibers, which means that HIIT can build more muscle than SST
- The intensity of the workouts can stimulate the release of muscle-building hormones, such as testosterone and growth hormone
- Generally burns more calories than SST, and so can produce weight-loss results similar to those of SST in a shorter period of time, with less risk of muscle loss
- Produces more of an "after-burn" effect than SST does

Note: Much has been made of the so-called after-burn effect, more technically known as **excess post-exercise oxygen consumption (EPOC)**. EPOC is a measurable increase in metabolic rate and oxygen consumption that can persist for several hours after a workout. The increases are part of the body's recovery process. The more intense the workout was, the longer the EPOC phase will be.

During EPOC, the body burns more calories than it would have done if the training had not occurred. However, the effect is actually very small, even after lengthy and very intense sessions of cardio. What's more, heavy weight training is now believed to produce a more significant after-burn effect than any type of cardio.

Disadvantages of interval training

- The intensity of the workouts, especially HIIT workouts, can be very stressful and difficult to maintain
- If overused, can lead to persistent stress- and anxiety-related symptoms, such as increased heart rate even while resting, difficulty sleeping, and an inability to relax and focus
- Easier to overtrain with interval training (especially HIIT) than it is with SST
- Higher risk of injury than there is with SST
- At very high intensities, rapidly depletes muscle glycogen stores. Once depleted, the body is more likely to use protein for energy, in which case there will be less protein available to repair muscle tissue damaged by exercise. This makes post-exercise protein consumption more important

Suitable exercises for interval training

Exercises and activities that are suitable for interval training include:

- Running
- Cycling
- Rowing
- Elliptical cross-training

Generally speaking, the other activities listed for SST are not suitable for interval training, especially HIIT, because they often can't produce and adequately maintain the required level of intensity. Arguably, the most ideal exercises for interval training are rowing and elliptical cross-training because they get your whole body involved while keeping the stress and impact on your joints to a minimum.

Circuit training

What is circuit training?

Like steady-state training, circuit training involves keeping your heart rate in a target training zone for a prescribed period of time. However, instead of using a single exercise or activity, such as jogging, you perform a series of different exercises with little to no rest between them. The exercises can include weight training exercises.

Applications of circuit training

Depending on the intensity of the exercises that you use, circuit training can help you to develop both aerobic and anaerobic metabolisms. However, generally speaking, it is less efficient than SST at developing aerobic metabolism and less efficient than interval training at developing anaerobic metabolism.

The main appeal of circuit training is that depending on the types of exercises that you use, it can help you to develop aspects of health and fitness that can't be developed using the other forms of cardio. For example, if you use plyometric exercises, you will develop the explosive abilities of your muscles and tendons, or if you use flexibility exercises, you will develop flexibility.

Note that even though you can use weight training exercises, circuit training can't be used to develop muscular size and strength beyond a low baseline. The reason is that it is not compatible with some of the important principles of effective weight training, such as muscle flushing and time under tension. What's more, weight training isolation exercises can't increase the heart rate to the desired levels. This is why weight training circuits have only been included in my beginner weight training programs, where they serve to promote neuromuscular adaptation and build muscular endurance.

Advantages of circuit training

- Can be used to develop a variety of aspects of fitness, from aerobic and anaerobic metabolism to speed, power, agility, flexibility, coordination, and balance
- Workouts can be designed around improving performance in specific sports
- Countless exercises to choose from, as well as numerous ways in which to structure the circuits and workouts
- Workouts can actually be fun!

Disadvantages of circuit training

- Depending on the exercises, there could be a high risk of injury
- Generally not as effective as SST and interval training at developing cardiorespiratory fitness and aerobic and anaerobic metabolisms

Suitable exercises for circuit training

Exercises that are suitable for circuit training include:

- Compound bodyweight exercises
- Compound free-weight exercises (including kettlebell exercises)
- Compound machine exercises
- Compound resistance band exercises
- Medicine ball and stability ball exercises
- Combat movements

In my opinion, the most beneficial types of exercises to use with circuit training are *functional* compound bodyweight exercises (for example, jumping jacks, burpees, mountain climbers, bear crawls, and squat jumps; see Table 14.1 at the end of the next chapter). Circuit training using such exercises is known as **functional circuit training (FCT)**.

As I have repeated throughout this book, functional strength is the kind of strength that is useful outside of the gym, in your everyday life. Functional compound bodyweight exercises are great for circuit training because they:

- can maintain your heart rate in the desired training zone
- are relatively safe
- don't require equipment
- are easy to transition between
- can often be adjusted to minimize their impact on joints
- can help you to develop functional strength and other aspects of fitness in addition to cardiorespiratory fitness.

Chapter 12: Cardio training programs

General instructions

Below I present three cardio training programs — one SST program (three workouts), one interval training program (three workouts), and one FCT program (two workouts). The workouts of the different training programs are interchangeable. In other words, you do not have to stick to a specific program; instead, you can complete any workout that you want to as long as you are suitable.

In addition to following a weight training program, complete 2 to 4 cardio workouts per week depending on your goal and preferences. For example, if you're cutting, you may want to complete up to 4 cardio workouts per week to help you to lose body fat, whereas if you're bulking, you may want to complete only 2 cardio workouts per week to keep improving cardiorespiratory fitness.

Remember that you need less cardio if your workouts are of a vigorous intensity and you need more cardio if your workouts are of a moderate intensity. Also, remember that compared with the long moderate-intensity workouts, the short vigorous-intensity workouts are generally more effective when trying to lose weight.

Keep the cardio workouts separate from your weight training workouts by at least a few hours. Performing the cardio workouts on your rest days is ideal. If you can't separate your cardio and weight training workouts, complete the weight training workouts before the cardio workouts.

If you're not following a weight training program, complete 3 to 5 cardio workouts per week, ideally, a mixture of SST, HIIT, and FCT.

The workouts have been categorized as either beginner, intermediate, or advanced. Beginner and intermediate workouts are aerobic; advanced workouts are either completely or partially anaerobic. Aerobic workouts, you are reminded, are below 85% maximum heart rate, whereas anaerobic workouts are 85% maximum heart rate and over.

If you're new to cardio, or if you've been away from cardio for over three months, please start with the beginner workouts, especially the beginner SST workout. From there, you can graduate to the other workouts in accordance with the progression guidelines. If you're experienced with cardio, you may start from a more suitable workout.

To monitor the progress of your cardiorespiratory fitness, every month or two, record your resting heart rate 30 to 60 minutes after exercise. With regular cardio, your post-exercise resting heart rate should reduce, indicating an improvement in fitness.

If you ever record an increase in resting heart rate, you are likely overusing the advanced workouts. In this case, please avoid the advanced workouts and emphasize the intermediate workouts to bring your resting heart rate down again.

Don't forget the importance of proper nutrition, especially when following both a weight training program and a cardio program. Remember that inadequate caloric intake and excessive SST cardio (or any type of aerobic training) can lead to muscle loss. The lengths of the aerobic workouts have been limited to 40 minutes to minimize this risk.

Every 6 to 12 weeks, take a break from cardio (especially if using HIIT) for a week to allow your system to recover. During this period, you should still keep active, though.

Steady-State Training (SST) Program

SST workout 1

- Suitability: Beginner
- Duration: 20–50 minutes including warmup and cooldown
- Training zone: Moderate (64%–76% HR_{max} or 40%–59% $HR_{reserve}$)
- Rate of perceived exertion (RPE): 12–13

Step 1

Start the selected exercise or activity at a slow pace or resistance and gradually increase your pace or resistance to build up to the target training zone or RPE by the end of 5 minutes.

Step 2

Maintain the target training zone or RPE for 10 to 40 minutes, depending on your abilities.

Step 3

Gradually reduce your pace or resistance and cool down for 5 minutes.

Progression

Once you can maintain Step 2 for 40 minutes, you can graduate to any of the intermediate workouts.

SST workout 2

- Suitability: Intermediate
- Duration: 20–50 minutes including warmup and cooldown
- Training zone: Vigorous, lower end (77%–84% HR_{max} or 60%–73% $HR_{reserve}$)
- RPE: 14–15

Step 1

Start the selected exercise or activity at a slow pace or resistance and gradually increase your pace or resistance to build up to the target training zone or RPE by the end of 5 minutes.

Step 2

Maintain the target training zone or RPE for 10 to 40 minutes, depending on your abilities.

Step 3

Gradually reduce your pace or resistance and cool down for 5 minutes.

Progression

Once you can maintain Step 2 for 40 minutes, you can graduate to any of the advanced workouts.

SST workout 3

- Suitability: Advanced
- Duration: 20–40 minutes including warmup and cooldown
- Training zone: Vigorous, upper end (85%–95% HR_{max} or 74%–89% $HR_{reserve}$)
- RPE: 16–17

Step 1

Start the selected exercise or activity at a slow pace or resistance and gradually increase your pace or resistance to build up to the target training zone or RPE by the end of 5 minutes.

Step 2

Maintain the target training zone or RPE for 10 to 30 minutes, depending on your abilities.

Step 3

Gradually reduce your pace or resistance and cool down for 5 minutes.

Interval Training Program

Interval training workout 1 (aerobic intervals in a 1:1 ratio)

- Suitability: Intermediate
- Equipment: Treadmill, exercise bike, rowing machine, or elliptical cross-trainer
- Duration: 28–46 minutes including warmup and cooldown
- Lower-intensity training zone: Moderate (64%–76% HR_{max} or 40%–59% $HR_{reserve}$)

- Lower-intensity RPE: 12–13
- Higher-intensity training zone: Vigorous, lower end (77%–84% HR_{max} or 60%–73% $HR_{reserve}$)
- Higher-intensity RPE: 14–15

Step 1

Start the selected exercise at a slow pace or resistance and gradually increase your pace or resistance to build up to the lower-intensity training zone or RPE by the end of 5 minutes.

Step 2

Alternate 3 minutes of training in the lower-intensity zone with 3 minutes of training in the higher-intensity zone. Do this 3 to 6 times.

Step 3

Gradually reduce your pace or resistance and cool down for 5 minutes.

Progression

Once you can easily complete Step 2 six times, you can graduate to any of the advanced workouts.

Interval training workout 2 (HIIT)

- Suitability: Advanced
- Equipment: Treadmill, exercise bike, rowing machine, or elliptical cross-trainer
- Duration: 28–37 minutes including warmup and cooldown
- Lower-intensity training zone: Moderate (64%–76% HR_{max} or 40%–59% $HR_{reserve}$)
- Lower-intensity RPE: 12–13
- Higher-intensity training zone: Near-maximal to maximal (≥96% HR_{max} or ≥90% $HR_{reserve}$)
- Higher-intensity RPE: 18–20

Step 1

Start the selected exercise at a slow pace or resistance and gradually increase your pace or resistance to build up to the lower-intensity training zone or RPE by the end of 5 minutes.

Step 2

Keep alternating between 4 minutes in the lower intensity training zone and 30 seconds in the higher intensity training zone. Do this 4 to 6 times. If you can do it more than 6 times, it means that you are not hitting a sufficiently high intensity during the 30-second intervals.

Step 3

Gradually reduce your pace or resistance and cool down for 5 minutes.

Interval training workout 3 (Tabata HIIT protocol)

- Suitability: Advanced
- Equipment: Treadmill, exercise bike, rowing machine, or elliptical cross-trainer
- Duration: Up to 14 minutes including warmup and cooldown
- Lower-intensity training zone: Light (57%–63% HR_{max} or 30%–39% $HR_{reserve}$)
- Lower-intensity RPE: 9–11
- Higher-intensity training zone: Near maximal or maximal (≥96% HR_{max} or ≥90% $HR_{reserve}$)
- Higher-intensity RPE: 18–20

Step 1

Choose your exercise and warm up for 5 minutes.

Step 2

Keep alternating between 20 seconds in the higher intensity training zone and 10 seconds in the lower intensity training zone. Do this a maximum of 8 times. If you can do it more than 8 times, it means that you are not hitting a sufficiently high intensity during the 20-second intervals.

Step 3

Gradually reduce your pace or resistance and cool down for 5 minutes.

Notes

If you use the treadmill with this protocol, you will have to stand on the edges during the 10-second recovery intervals.

The Tabata protocol is probably the most famous HIIT regimen. It was originally published in 1996 by Professor Izumi Tabata and colleagues. The protocol had been designed to train speed skaters. Professor Tabata had tested it in an experiment and compared the results with the results of an SST experiment, both of which involved amateur athletes and a cycle ergometer (an exercise bike that can measure exercise intensity).

In the SST experiment, the athletes performed moderate-intensity SST for 60 minutes a day, 5 days a week, for 6 consecutive weeks. The researchers found that the athletes showed an improvement in aerobic capacity of 9.5% and, as expected, no improvement in anaerobic capacity.

In the Tabata experiment, the athletes used the Tabata protocol for 5 days a week, for 6 consecutive weeks. The researchers found that the athletes showed improvements in both aerobic capacity of 14% and anaerobic capacity of 28%. In other words, the four-minute maximal-intensity Tabata workouts had produced both anaerobic benefits and similar aerobic benefits to doing sixty-minute moderate-intensity SST workouts! The results were pretty shocking at the time, indicating that you could get both aerobic and anaerobic benefits from only a four-minute (albeit extremely intense) workout.

If you're going to follow the Tabata protocol, please get clearance from your healthcare professional first. Do not use it for more than 5 days a week, and take a week off from it after 6 weeks. Remember that it's designed to improve the performance of professional athletes.

Functional Circuit Training (FCT) Program

FCT workout 1

- Suitability: Beginner
- Equipment: None
- Duration: 24–39 minutes including warmup and cooldown
- Training zone: Moderate (64%–76% HR_{max} or 40%–59% $HR_{reserve}$)
- RPE: 12–13

Step 1

Warm up with five minutes of dynamic stretching.

Step 2

Complete each step of Circuit 1 twice. Move between the steps without resting. If you feel up to it, once you complete the circuit, take a 1-minute break and then repeat the circuit.

Step	Primary exercise (40 seconds)	Active rest (20 seconds)
1	Bodyweight squat	Jog on the spot
2	Walking lunge	Upper cuts
3	Side shuffle	Standing walkout plank
4	Mountain climber	Push-up on knees
5	Bicycle crunch	Lying side hip raise
6	Bear crawl	Plank with rotation
7	Burpee	Duck walk

Circuit 1. Functional bodyweight exercises.

Step 3

Cool down with five minutes of dynamic stretching.

Progression

Once completing two circuits becomes easy, you can graduate to any of the intermediate workouts.

FCT workout 2

- Suitability: Intermediate
- Equipment: Dumbbells
- Duration: 39 minutes including warmup and cooldown
- Target training zone: Vigorous, lower end (77%–84% HR_{max} or 60%–73% $HR_{reserve}$)
- RPE: 14–15

Step 1

Warm up with five minutes of dynamic stretching.

Step 2

Complete each step of Circuit 2 twice. Move between the steps without resting. Once you have completed the circuit, take a 1-minute break and then repeat the circuit.

Step	Primary exercise (40 seconds)	Active rest (20 seconds)
1	Squat jump	Boxer's shuffle
2	Jumping lunge	Dumbbell wood chop
3	Dumbbell Romanian deadlift	Bent-over two-arm dumbbell row
4	Push-up with dumbbell row	Crab crawl
5	Lying leg and hip raise	Russian twist
6	Break dancer	Lying oblique twist
7	Single-leg burpee	Inch worm

Circuit 2. Functional bodyweight and dumbbell exercises.

Step 3

Cool down with five minutes of dynamic stretching.

224

Progression

Once completing Step 2 becomes easy, you can graduate to any of the advanced workouts.

How to design your own FCT workouts

Primary and active rest exercises

Designing your own FCT workouts is easy!

As you can see from the FCT workouts that I have provided, each step of a circuit consists of two exercises:

1. A primary exercise, performed for 40 seconds
2. An active rest exercise, performed for 20 seconds

The purpose of the primary exercises, which are of a higher intensity than the active rest exercises, is to get your heart racing. The purpose of the active rest exercises is to allow you to momentarily catch your breath before the next primary exercise, while also keeping you moving (hence "active" rest).

Step-by-step procedure

With that in mind, to design your own FCT workouts, just follow this procedure:

1. Choose some primary and active rest exercises from Table 14.1. The active rest exercises are presented in italic type.
2. Match each primary exercise with a suitable active rest exercise. There are fewer active rest exercises, so you will have to repeat some.
3. Arrange the matches into a list, and you will have your own FCT circuit!

Note that the primary and active rest exercises presented in Table 14.1 are just a small sample selection. There are numerous suitable exercises out there for you to choose from. If you have a stability ball, a medicine ball, and/or resistance bands, the number of exercises at your disposal will be absolutely huge! As mentioned in the previous chapter, you can also use combat movements, compound free-weight exercises, and compound machine exercises, such as roundhouse kicks, seated cable rows, barbell deadlifts, and dumbbell squats.

General guidelines

As you design your circuits, keep the following in mind.

- You can make your circuits as long as you want, provided they can keep your heartbeat in the target training zone for 10–40 minutes.

- Try to incorporate all types of movement patterns (squatting, lunging, flexing/extending the hips, bending sideways, twisting the torso, pulling, pushing, jogging, and jumping).
- Try to incorporate both bilateral (two-sided) and unilateral (one-sided) exercises.
- Try to incorporate exercises that promote agility, speed, power, flexibility, coordination, and balance.
- Select exercises that are easy to transition between.
- Favor exercises that subject your joints to the lowest level of impact.
- Avoid exercises that could be dangerous.
- As always, learn how to perform the exercises with optimal form so as to prevent injuries and get the most out of them. You should be able to find instructions and videos for some of the exercises on my website, **weighttraining.guide**. For the rest, please check YouTube.

Whole body	Lower body	Upper body	Core
Jumping jack	Bodyweight squat	Chest dip	Bicycle crunch
Fly jack	Pistol squat	Push-up with rotation	Leg and hip raise
Lizard hop	Squat jack	Diamond push-up	Hanging wipers
Burpee	Squat jump	Plyo push-up	Sit-up
Single-leg burpee	Broad jump	Pike push-up	Jack-knife sit-up
Bear crawl	Star jump	Pike press	V-up
Single-leg bear crawl	Tuck jump	Spiderman push-up	Hyperextension
Gorilla crawl	Skater jump	Pull-up	Plank jack
Table top crawl	High-knee run	L-sit pull-up	Plank jump-in
Break dancer	Butt kicks	Chin-up	*Plank with rotation*
Get-ups	Shuttle run	L-sit chin-up	*Plank shoulder tap*
Superman push-up	Carioca quick step Side	Muscle up	*Plank knee tap*
Standing walkout plank	shuffle	*Push-up on knees*	*Plank roll*
Inch worm	Lunge	*Self-assisted pull-up*	*Lying heel touch*
Baby crawl	Curtsy lunge	*Inverted row*	*Lying side hip raise*
Crab crawl	Jumping lunge	*Triceps dip*	*Lying oblique twist*
Lateral crab crawl	Step-up	*Scissor chops*	*Russian twist*
Plank crawl	Side/Front kicks	*Boxer's hooks*	*Reverse crunch*
Bird dog	*Duck walk*	*Upper cuts*	*Superman*
	Glute bridge	*Jab crosses*	*Dead bug*
	Good morning		
	Flutter kick		
	Leg raise		
	Donkey kick		

Table 14.1. Primary and active rest functional bodyweight exercises categorized by body region. Active rest exercises are presented in italic type and have been chosen arbitrarily based on the assumption that they should be easier than the other exercises for most people. You may of course differentiate between your own primary and active rest exercises based on your personal abilities and preferences.

PART 6: WEIGHT LOSS GUIDE

Chapter 13: Three steps to easier and permanent weight loss

Introduction to the Weight Loss Guide

As many people know too well, losing weight can be very difficult. What's more, if you manage to lose weight, keeping it off can be even more difficult!

In this short guide, I reveal three steps and a broad range of tips that can make losing weight, and keeping it off permanently, much easier. The permanent weight loss is still going to be a challenge, but it's going to be far less of a challenge, which means that your chances of succeeding will be significantly increased. First, let's go over a few key points about weight loss.

Key points

1. The formula for losing weight is simple

Your body needs a certain number of kilocalories each day to fuel your bodily functions and physical activities. In order to lose weight, each day, all you have to do is consume fewer kilocalories than your body needs.

That's it. That really is the gist of weight loss. As long as you eat fewer kilocalories than your body needs, you will lose weight — even if you only eat chocolate!

2. Not all kilocalories are equal

Even though you can eat nothing but chocolate and still lose weight, you obviously must never do such a thing. To promote optimal health, you must primarily consume nutrient-dense foods that provide your body with everything it needs for survival, growth, and repair. As you'll learn below, this certainly does not mean that you have to struggle through boring meals every day.

3. Some foods make weight loss much more difficult

The foods that you eat can affect your metabolism. Some "healthy" foods can slow down your metabolism and make weight loss much more difficult. They can even encourage your body to store fat! Other foods can speed up your metabolism and encourage your body to burn fat. Knowing what foods to eat and what foods to avoid can therefore make losing weight much easier. More on this in Step two.

4. To keep the weight off, you must enjoy your new diet

Probably the biggest challenge to losing weight and keeping it off is the temptation to return to your old diet. The new diet is usually alien, tasteless, depressing, and lacks diversity, which makes you yearn for your old favorite dishes and delicacies. In order to stick to a new diet, it must include a wide range of easy-to-prepare meals that excite you, keep you feeling full, and make you happy, in addition to providing you with everything you need for health and wellbeing.

5. *To preserve your muscle mass when you diet, you must lift weights*

When you diet and put your body into a state of caloric deficit, your body can burn your muscles for fuel if it thinks that they are not being used. Initially, it burns glycogen stores in your liver, before moving on to fat stores. However, it doesn't like using up fat stores because fat is a rich source of energy, so the body soon turns to unused muscle mass. Loss of muscle is not a bad thing only if you're a guy but also if you're a girl because muscle is what gives you your shape and curves. If you lose muscle and then put all of the fat back on again, your body will look less shapely and toned than it did before losing the muscle. The best way to avoid losing muscle mass when you diet is to lift weights, which will tell your body that your muscles are in use and important.

6. *Rapid weight loss is not good for you*

If you do manage to lose weight, it's very important that you do not lose weight too quickly. The reason is that rapid weight loss increases your likelihood of losing muscle mass, even if you lift weights. What's more, if you were significantly overweight, rapid weight loss could leave you with ugly, loose skin. In extreme cases, rapid weight loss can even damage your liver!

The three steps

Now that I've laid down those key points, I can reveal the three steps to successful and permanent weight loss. As you will notice, the three steps address the concerns raised in the key points.

Step one

Install MyFitnessPal on your phone. (If you don't have a phone, you can use the MyFitnessPal website, which provides the same functionalities.) The app and website are free. Once you set up the app, it will tell you how many kilocalories you have to eat each day to lose weight. You're going to add everything you eat and drink to the app, and it's going to count your kilocalories for you. It's also going to show you if you're getting enough of the right macronutrients, vitamins, and minerals, which is useful if you want to be healthy. Adding your meals is easier than you think, and the process becomes increasingly easier the more you use the app. All you have to do is consume the number of kilocalories the app asks you to consume, and you will lose weight. It's as simple as that. I explain how to set up the app for successful weight loss at the end of this guide.

Note that you will not have to count kilocalories for the rest of your life. After several months of using the app to count your kilocalories, you will learn portion sizes and portion control, after which you can stop counting kilocalories and use portion size estimates.

Step two

Download the Metabolic Cooking package:

http://weighttraining.guide/go/cookingpackage/

The package will make losing weight, and keeping it off, much easier, not to mention tastier. The package includes a cookbook that contains 250 genuinely tasty, nutrient-dense, and easy-to-prepare recipes (breakfasts, dinners, lunches, desserts, sides, snacks, and smoothies). The recipes are designed to boost your metabolism and encourage your body to burn fat. The package also includes various guides that will teach you everything you need to know about tasty fat-loss cooking, including what ingredients encourage your body to store fat and what ingredients help your body to burn fat. You will never again have to struggle through bland weight loss meals that bore you to tears! Instead, you'll be able to enjoy tasty and exciting fat-burning meals that will make you happy, boost your energy levels, and keep you feeling full for longer. This in turn will increase your likelihood of sticking to your diet and keeping the weight off. Best of all, the whole package only costs $10.

Step three

Start training. As you're aware, weight training is important to preserve your muscles and shape, and cardio can help you to lose the weight. In this book, you have more than enough training program and workout options to choose from. Take advantage of them.

Remember, the minimalistic weight training program together with just two short steady-state cardio workouts per week are enough to completely transform your body — from muscles to heart and lungs — and dramatically improve your weight, body composition, health, fitness, athleticism, and appearance. Try them. Once you start seeing results, you will almost certainly want to move on to the more advanced weight training and cardio programs.

Additional tips for easier weight loss

Here are some additional tips that should be useful in promoting successful and permanent weight loss. The tips will help you to be more active, overcome urges to break your diet, feel full for longer, avoid overeating, and keep motivated and committed to your goal of losing weight.

Stay active

In addition to training, there are lots of other ways in which you could increase your activity level and thus boost the number of kilocalories that you burn each day. Some of these methods can actually be quite enjoyable. For example, you could:

- go for a walk every night and listen to an audiobook
- cycle through parks or nature reserves
- join a swimming club
- start martial arts or yoga
- take up a sport, such as tennis, squash, or soccer

- take up a physical hobby, such as dancing
- frequently go hiking or camping.

Other ways in which you could increase your activity level include the following.

- Use an exercise bike or strider as you watch TV
- Work on foot by placing a platform on your desk
- Sit on a stability ball instead of a chair at work
- Stop taking the car everywhere you go
- Get off the bus/train one stop early and walk the rest of the way
- Take the stairs instead of the elevator
- Go for a brisk walk during your lunch breaks

Put your weight loss goal into writing

One effective way of making your weight loss mission official and reducing your chances of breaking your diet is to put it into writing. Sign and date it, and stick it on your fridge. Even better, get a loved one to sign it as well. Whenever you feel the urge to break your diet, you will see the signed and dated "contract" on your fridge, which will make breaking your diet much more difficult.

Occupy yourself if urges strike

Whenever you have a strong urge to break your diet, find something to keep your mind occupied for a few minutes. For example, take a shower, call a friend, or play a videogame. In most cases, simply taking your mind off food for just a few moments can allow your urges to subside, after which you will have more control of yourself.

Don't give up if you mess up

If you break your diet on occasions — and you almost certainly will — do not lose enthusiasm and give up. This kind of all-or-nothing mentality is foolish. Messing up on occasions is normal and doesn't spell the end of your weight loss mission. Accept the glitch and carry on. Don't let it ruin all previous successful days of sticking to your diet. If you want to, you can make up for the glitch by eating slightly less in your next couple of meals.

Make sure to get lots of protein and fiber

Compared with fat and carbohydrate, protein keeps you feeling full for longer, which reduces your chances of succumbing to urges and breaking your diet. Fiber, too, can help you feel full for longer. Therefore, get lots of protein and fiber in each meal. As to fat and carbohydrate, the former keeps you feeling full for longer than the latter.

Use smaller plates and glasses

The larger your plate is, the larger your serving size is likely to be. Simply using smaller plates and glasses can dramatically reduce the sizes of your portions/servings and thus your caloric intake.

Limit variety during mealtimes

If you cook a bunch of different things for a meal, you're likely to have a bit of each one. Therefore, limit variety when you cook. For example, you don't need both potatoes and sweet potatoes when you make a roast; sweet potatoes should suffice.

Eat slowly

As you eat, it takes 15 to 20 minutes for your stomach to tell your brain that you're full, which makes it easy to overeat if you eat quickly. If you slow down your eating, you'll find yourself feeling full before you eat as much food as you usually would.

Chew gum

Try chewing sugar-free gum if you're still hungry after a meal, or if you get hungry before it's time for a meal. Gum helps many people to stop overeating and/or cope with cravings. Note, however, that too much gum can have laxative and other negative effects, so choose your gum carefully, and don't overdo it.

Join weight loss forums

At any moment in time, numerous people are trying to lose weight. They're all going through the same challenging process as you are. You'll find many thousands of them in online forums, where they support, guide, and motivate each other. Join a few such weight loss forums and make friends. Share your goals, achievements, and journey. The journey is easier with companions.

Allow yourself a weekly cheat meal

If you stick to your diet, reward yourself with a cheat meal at the end of the week. The cheat meal will not affect your progress. What it will do is help you a great deal to stay motivated and committed to your goal of losing weight.

Use social media for weight loss help and motivation

- Join Meetup.com and attend weight loss meetups to make friends, share your journey, and receive encouragement.
- Start a weight loss blog and document your weight loss journey. Your journey will motivate your readership, and your readership will keep you motivated with encouragement. You can also monetize your blog.
- Start a YouTube channel and document your weight loss journey using videos. As with a blog, you can help your viewers, and they will help you with encouragement. You can also make money from your videos through the YouTube Partner Program.

- Subscribe to the YouTube channels of others who are documenting their own weight loss journey, learn from them, and be motivated by their success stories.
- Start an Instagram account and document your weight loss journey using photos and short videos. The encouragement offered by your followers will help you on your way to losing weight.

How to set up MyFitnessPal for successful weight loss

Let's now go over how to set up MyFitnessPal for successful and healthy weight loss. The process doesn't actually need much explaining; setting up MyFitnessPal is quite straightforward.

Setting up the account

During the process of setting up your MyFitnessPal account, whether you do it on your phone or on the website, you'll be asked for your personal details, goals, and activity level.

- Your personal details are your height, current weight, gender, and date of birth.
- Your goals are your weekly goal (how much weight you want to lose per week) and your goal weight (the weight you are ultimately aiming for).
- Your activity level is the amount of activity that you undertake in an average day, not including any exercises or physical activities outside of your job.

For your weekly goal, choose "Lose 1 lb per week". I realize that this isn't much, and you probably want to lose more; however, this is the recommended amount if you want to avoid losing weight too quickly. Remember, if you lose weight too quickly, you will also lose muscle and may even end up with ugly, loose skin. For the first couple of weeks, you'll probably lose more than one pound per week anyway — especially if you're significantly overweight. That's fine. The amount you lose should soon settle down.

When you select your goal weight, be realistic, and start with a simple goal. That way, you'll be much more likely to achieve it and feel encouraged. For example, if you currently weigh 210 pounds, make your goal weight 205 pounds, which is easily achievable. Once you achieve your first goal, you can change your goal weight to 200 pounds and start your second goal.

Once you enter all of the necessary information into MyFitnessPal, the app will calculate the number of kilocalories you have to eat each day to achieve your weekly goal. All you have to do is add to your diary the meals that you consume and the exercises and activities that you perform. The more exercises and physical activities you add, the more kilocalories you will be able to eat!

How to add your meals and exercises

I explain how to add your meals and exercises to MyFitnessPal in the **Nutrition Guide**, in **How to track your calories and diet**. Just remember that you have to add *everything* that you eat and drink (except water, which is optional). This includes alcoholic beverages, dressings, seasonings, and condiments, the kilocalories of which can really add up.

Increase the protein ratio to avoid losing muscle

After you have set up MyFitnessPal, you can adjust the ratio of macronutrients (carbohydrate, fat, and protein) that you have to eat in the Goals section of the app. The default ratio is 50% carbohydrate, 30% fat, and 20% protein.

To reduce your likelihood of losing much muscle as you lose weight, increase the protein ratio to 30% or even 35%. The extra protein in your system will ensure that your body has enough protein to rebuild muscle tissues that are broken down for energy.

After adjusting your protein ratio, you will also have to adjust the ratios of carbohydrate and fat to ensure that they collectively equal 100%. I leave you to decide what percentages to choose based on your preferences. Keep in mind that, as revealed in the *2015–2020 Dietary Guidelines for Americans*, the US Department of Agriculture recommends the following daily ranges for men and women aged 19 and over:

- Carbohydrate: 45%–65% of kilocalories
- Fat: 20%–35% of kilocalories
- Protein: 10%–35% of kilocalories

Keep MyFitnessPal updated

In addition to adding your meals and exercises to MyFitnessPal, every couple of weeks, you have to update your current weight to inform MyFitnessPal of your progress. The app will then recalculate your caloric needs and ensure that you keep losing weight. If you don't update your current weight and keep consuming the same number of kilocalories per day, your weight loss will slow down and stop.

Note that whenever you edit your current weight, MyFitnessPal resets your custom settings, so you will have to re-adjust your macronutrient ratio settings if you changed them.

ABOUT THE AUTHOR

My name's Edward Lord. Although my background is in paleobiology, I've been a medical writer and editor since 2006. I've also been a bodybuilding and fitness enthusiast since I was a child.

Born and raised in London, I have trained on and off since the age of nine, sometimes producing what some people might call a great body. I've also gone through periods where I have become lazy and put on lots of weight. At my heaviest, in my early thirties, I weighed 231 pounds, much of which was fat. After getting diagnosed with mild non-alcoholic fatty liver disease, I pulled my act together and got back into shape, where I have remained into my late thirties.

I love bodybuilding and fitness probably more than anyone I have ever met. After all these years, I still get a buzz when I train, and I can never wait to get back into the gym. I love the gym lifestyle and culture, and I especially love the feeling that I get after a workout, as I leave the gym with my joints feeling well-oiled and my muscles feeling like they're about to explode!

Another thing that I love is learning about fitness and bodybuilding. As someone with a strong background in life sciences, my research goes much deeper than average. I like to understand everything at a deep scientific level so that when I train, I do it properly.

For me, training isn't just about building muscle and strength. I also understand the importance of improving my endurance, agility, flexibility, balance, coordination, posture, gait, muscle strength ratios, and body composition. Only then can you truly have a great body.

This book contains everything you need to create a great body. I researched it thoroughly, wrote it with care, and did my best to explain everything as clearly as possible. No matter what your fitness goal is, I sincerely hope that it helps you to achieve it.

Edward Lord

P.S.

I'll be very grateful if you write a review of my book on Amazon.

For further assistance, see my website and social media pages

- **Website:** weighttraining.guide
- **Instagram:** instagram.com/weighttrainingguide/
- **Facebook:** facebook.com/officialweighttrainingguide/
- **Pinterest:** pinterest.com/weighttrainingg/
- **YouTube:** youtube.com/c/WeighttrainingGuide

Made in the USA
Middletown, DE
29 October 2020